D1191709

Smith's Recognizable Patterns of Human Deformation

SECOND EDITION

John M. Graham, Jr., M.D., Sc.D.

Director, Clinical Genetics and Dysmorphology Program
Associate Professor, Maternal and Child Health
Dartmouth Medical School
Hanover, New Hampshire

1988   **W. B. SAUNDERS COMPANY**
Harcourt Brace Jovanovich, Inc.

Philadelphia • London • Toronto • Montreal • Sydney • Tokyo

W. B. SAUNDERS COMPANY
Harcourt Brace Jovanovich, Inc.

The Curtis Center
Independence Square West
Philadelphia, PA 19106

Library of Congress Cataloging-in-Publication Data

Smith, David W., 1926–1981.
  Smith's recognizable patterns of human deformation.

  Rev. ed. pf: Recognizable patterns of human deformation/by
David W. Smith.   1981.
Includes bibliographical references and index.

1. Abnormalities, Human—Etiology.   2. Human
    mechanics.   3. Morphogenesis.   4. Birth injuries.
5. Growth disorders.   I. Graham, John M., 1947–
II. Title. [DNLM: 1. Abnormalities.   2. Biomechanics.
QS 675 S644r]

RG627.5.S57   616'.043   88–18316

ISBN 0–7216–2338–7

Editor: Lisette Bralow

Developmental Editor: Linda Mills

Designer: Karen O'Keefe

Production Manager: Peter Faber

Manuscript Editor: Ruth Low

Illustration Coordinator: Brett MacNaughton

Page Layout Artist: Dorothy Chattin

Indexer: William Cole

Smith's Recognizable Patterns of Human Deformation   ISBN 0–7216–2338–7

Last digit is the print number: 9   8   7   6   5   4   3   2

Dedication
(to the second edition)

To Lyle M. Harrah
Dysmorphology Research Librarian

A major contributor to all of Dr. Smith's books,
for years, she has provided his fellows and colleagues
with a weekly Dysmorphology Reading List.

Acknowledgments

In the acknowledgment section of the first edition of this book, which was published in 1981, Dr. Smith wrote: "It was February 1975, at an international meeting on nomenclature for birth defects, that I first heard Peter Dunn, M.D., of Bristol, England, give his impassioned plea for a clear distinction between defects due to mechanical constraint forces (deformation) as contrasted to those due to poor formation (malformation). . . . Since that time I have been ever more impressed by the importance, relevance, and magnitude of this deformational category of birth defects. Hence, I acknowledge Peter Dunn as the individual who set me forth on the pathway that culminated in this book."

While I was a fellow with Dr. Smith from 1978 to 1980, we investigated many of the concepts set forth in this book. This effort was greatly helped by Dr. Smith's previous fellows, to whom he dedicated the first edition of this book. Dr. Smith's dysmorphology fellows (listed in chronologic order) were Drs. John Opitz, Luc Lemli, Bob Summitt, Jules LeRoy, Arlan Rosenbloom, Jaime Frias, Jon Aase, Bryan Hall, Kenneth Lyons Jones, James Hanson, Sterling Clarren, Marvin Miller, Albert Schinzel, John M. Graham, Jr., and Margot VanAllen. Drs. Judy Hall and Mike Cohen also helped to collect and to disseminate much of the information contained in *Recognizable Patterns of Human Deformation*. After completing the first edition of this book and the revision of its companion text, *Recognizable Patterns of Human Malformation* (1982), Dr. Smith died on January 21, 1981. He requested that I continue his work and revise this book.

Many of the photographs were taken by Dr. Smith's research associate, Ms. Mary Ann Sedgewick Harvey, and most of the medical illustrations were prepared by Ms. Phyllis Wood of the University of Washington Health Sciences Learning Resource Center. Dr. Kate Donahue provided many of the anthropological observations as part of a Saul Blatman Clinical Fellowship Award.

Mrs. Lyle M. Harrah has continued to provide references and a host of background literature for this revised edition. Dr. Dave Smith found her of "inestimable value" and greatly appreciated "her dedication and capacity for obtaining even the most obscure reference." Her many years of service to Dr. Smith continue to this day as she enters her ninth decade. She has faithfully compiled and distributed the Dysmorphology Reading List to Dr. Smith's many fellows, friends, and colleagues. We acknowledge her astonishing energy by dedicating this book to Lyle M. Harrah.

Contents

1

Introduction

Mechanical forces play an important role in both normal and abnormal morphogenesis. Anomalies that represent the normal response of a tissue to unusual mechanical forces are termed *deformations,* in contrast to *malformations,* which denote a primary problem in the morphogenesis of a tissue, and *disruptions,* which represent the breakdown of a previously normal tissue (Fig. 1–1). There are predominantly two types of deformation problems: those in which the causative forces were due to an intrinsic problem of the fetus,* such as a malformation, and those in which the deformation was produced by mechanical forces that were extrinsic to an otherwise normal fetus (Figs. 1–2 and 1–3).

Additional examples of intrinsic deformations secondary to a malformation are considered in Chapter 4. This text is primarily concerned with *extrinsic deformations* produced by constraint in utero of an otherwise normal fetus. Extrinsic forces may cause a single localized deformation, such as a deformed foot, or they may cause a deformation sequence. A deformation sequence refers to the manifold molding effects of a given deforming situation. A good example is the oligohydramnios sequence, in which oligohydramnios is responsible for a number of deformations. The single deformations are presented in atlas form along with the deformation sequences. The major cause of such

deformations is uterine constraint of the rapidly growing malleable fetus in late gestation as the fetus tends to outgrow the uterus. Most of the molded deformations have an excellent prognosis, once the fetus is released from the constraining environment. However, some of them merit treatment, and this usually involves the use of gentle mechanical forces to attempt to *reshape* the anomaly to a more normal form.

A clear distinction between deformation and malformation is critical to providing the parents with a clear understanding of the problem and its prognosis, management, and recurrence risk. In general, the prognosis is *much* more favorable if the problem is deformation rather than malformation. The collective frequency of extrinsic deformations of late fetal origin, such as those set forth in Chapter Two, is about 2 per cent of liveborn babies.[1] Hence, this text deals with common problems.

A broader clinical approach toward the problems of deformation is presented in Chapter Three, and the basic principles of biomechanics plus the role of mechanical factors in the normal as well as abnormal morphogenesis of particular tissues are set forth in Chapter Four.

Reference

1. Dunn, P. M.: The influence of the intrauterine environment in the causation of congenital postural deformities, with special reference to congenital dislocation of the hip. (Thesis for M. D. degree.) University of Cambridge, 1969.

---

*The embryo and fetus are collectively referred to as the fetus in this text. Fetus in Latin basically means "the young one."

Types of Problems in
MORPHOGENESIS

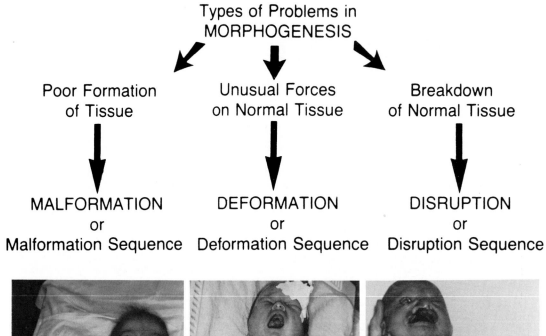

Poor Formation
of Tissue

Unusual Forces
on Normal Tissue

Breakdown
of Normal Tissue

MALFORMATION
or
Malformation Sequence

DEFORMATION
or
Deformation Sequence

DISRUPTION
or
Disruption Sequence

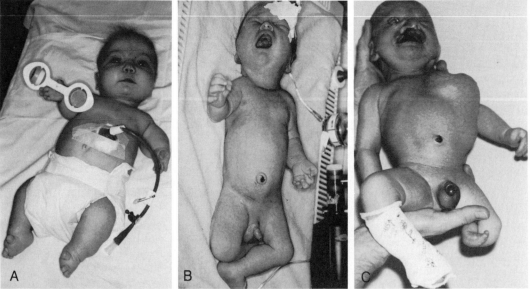

A   B   C

Figure 1–1. The three major types of problems in morphogenesis are demonstrated here. On the left *(A)* is an infant with diastrophic dysplasia, which results in multiple joint contractures due to abnormal connective tissue. The infant in the center *(B)* experienced prolonged oligohydramnios from 17 weeks' gestation until birth. The infant on the right *(C)* demonstrates limb and body wall defects that resulted from disruption after early amnion rupture and localized limb and body wall hemorrhages.

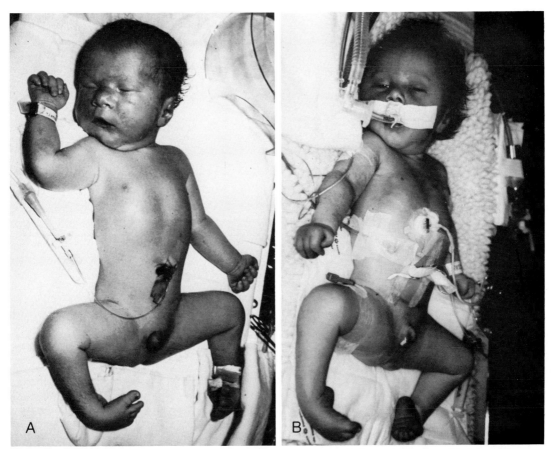

Figure 1–2. Examples of intrinsic deformation. *A,* Congenital myotonic dystrophy. *B,* Pena-Shokeir syndrome.

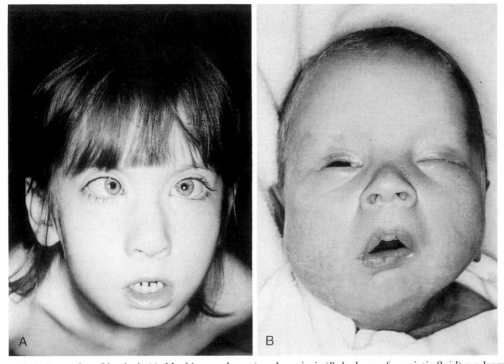

Figure 1–3. Examples of intrinsic (*A,* Moebius syndrome) and extrinsic (*B,* leakage of amniotic fluid) syndromes.

Patterns of Deformation

1.0 JOINT CONTRACTURE, ESPECIALLY OF THE FOOT

GENERAL. Any cause of prolonged immobilization of a joint tends to give rise to joint fixation with contracture. This can result from immobilization due to external constraint, from intrinsic neuromuscular problems, or from defects in the formation of the joint and/or its connective tissue, as summarized in Figures 2–1 through 2–2. When the problem is the result of external constraint, the position of a given joint reflects the nature of the forces that resulted in the deformation. The most common region affected is the foot, though fixations of other joints may also occur. When there are fixations of multiple joints the term *arthrogryposis* is utilized (Fig. 2–1). This term designates a category and *not* a diagnosis.

According to Ruth Wynne-Davies,[1] congenital malposition of the foot, often loosely referred to as *clubfoot*, occurs with a frequency of about 4 per 1000 births. Probably more than half of these represent deformations due to external constraint in utero. The prognosis is much better for this constraint category than for any of the other causes of joint contracture.

Evaluation of the foot includes determining the full range of its mobility. Roentgenograms are of little value in early infancy because the bones are not sufficiently ossified to allow for the relevant assessment. Among the associated anomalies that tend to occur with *postural* equinovarus or calcaneovalgus types of foot deformities are joint laxity

Table 2–1. **METHODS OF MANAGEMENT FOR FOOT CONTRACTURE**

Method	Comment
Manual stretching, toward normal form	Performed at each feeding and diaper change
Adhesive taping, toward normal form	This method is gaining in popularity. Use tincture of benzoin to protect the skin
Splinting	Devices such as the Denis-Browne splint and reversed-last shoes may be utilized, especially at night, to maintain desired position
Plaster cast	Though casting may be utilized to correct position, it is best used to maintain an improved form that has been achieved by manipulation, taping, and/or surgery
Surgery	If more conservative measures have not resulted in improvement of foot position during early infancy, surgery merits consideration. The present tendency is to operate earlier on resistant cases, including those that are secondary to a neurologic problem

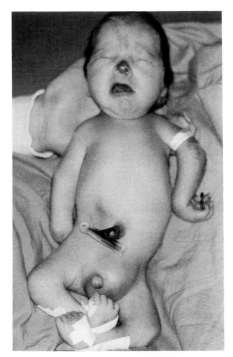

Figure 2–1. This infant has the amyoplasia form of arthrogryposis, a sporadic condition attributed to spinal cord damage (possibly with a vascular basis) in early gestation. Fetal movement is limited, with joint ankylosis and absent flexion creases. The posture of this condition is quite characteristic, with the hands fixed in external rotation and extension of the elbows (the "policeman's tip" position). This would be an example of intrinsic deformation due to vascular disruption.

(10 per cent) and inguinal hernia (7 per cent). These findings suggest that minor connective tissue problems may enhance the liability to positional deformation of the foot. The postural deformities that have had their onset in utero may be perpetuated by particular sleeping postures in early infancy. Hence, consideration of sleeping posture and whether it is, or is not, augmenting the deformation may be an important part of the evaluation.

A number of modes of management have been utilized in attempts to restore the foot to its usual position.[2] These are summarized in Table 2–1. Alteration of sleeping posture is another consideration. Each type of foot contracture should be considered individually, as to both prognosis and management. For example, the prognosis for calcaneovalgus with manipulative stretching alone is usually excellent, whereas about half of the cases of equinovarus contracture resist correction by conservative measures. This is one of the many reasons why I believe the term clubfoot should be eliminated.

References

1. Wynne-Davies, R.: Family studies and aetiology of club foot. J. Med. Genet. 2:227, 1965.
2. Lloyd-Roberts, G. C.: Orthopaedics in Infancy and Childhood. New York, Appleton-Century-Crofts, 1971.

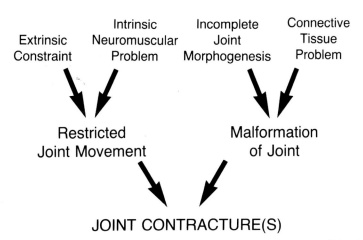

Figure 2–2. Joint contracture at birth may be the consequence of a number of modes of developmental pathology, of which in-utero constraint is the most common.

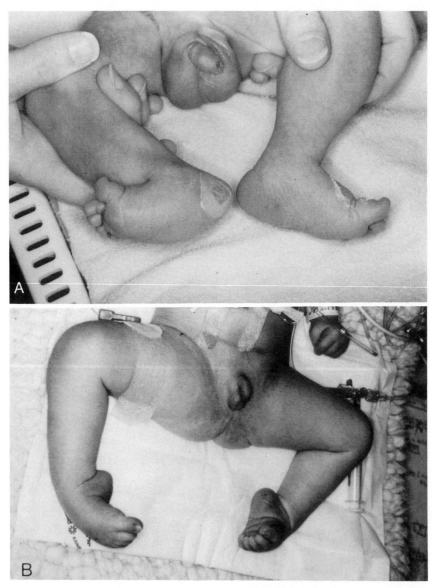

Figure 2–3. *A,* This infant has bilateral equinovarus foot deformations due to prolonged oligohydramnios resulting from leaking amniotic fluid from 17 weeks' gestation until birth. This is an example of extrinsic deformation. *B,* This infant with Type 1 Pena-Shokeir syndrome demonstrates bilateral equinovarus foot deformities due to fetal akinesia deformation sequence (intrinsic deformation).

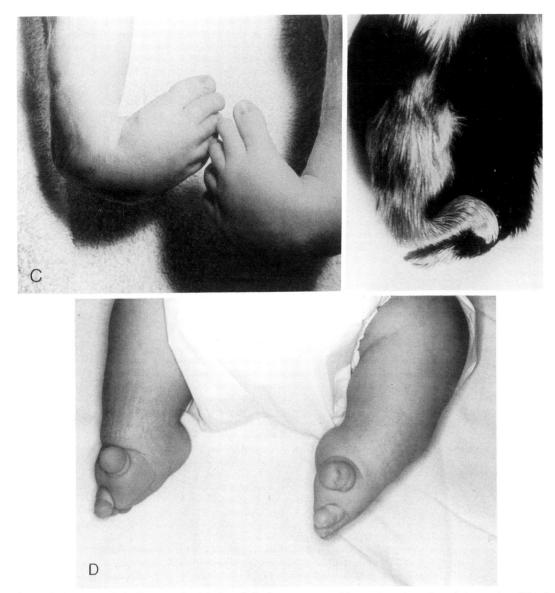

Figure 2–3 *Continued. C,* Neurogenic club feet (left) due to maternal hyperthermia at 4 weeks' gestation. This is also demonstrated in the guinea pig on the right, which was born to a mother exposed to hyperthermia in an incubator during early gestation (also an example of intrinsic deformation). *D,* These equinovarus feet resulted from a connective tissue abnormality in an infant with diastrophic dysplasia. This is an example of a connective tissue dysplasia giving rise to malformation of a joint.

1.1 Calcaneovalgus

(Dorsiflexed Foot)

GENESIS. This deformity, which has a frequency of 1 per 1000 births,[1] is most commonly the result of uterine constraint having forced the foot into a dorsiflexed position against the lower leg. It is especially common with extended legs following prolonged breech position. Partly for this reason, it has a non-random association with dislocation of the hip. Dislocation of the hip, which is found in 5 per cent of patients with calcaneovalgus,[1] obviously merits high risk consideration in any newborn with this foot deformity. Calcaneovalgus is more common in firstborn infants and about four times more common in females than in males.[1] This latter observation may relate to the greater degree of joint laxity in females than in males. In keeping with this hypothesis, there is an increased frequency (10 per cent) of joint laxity in first degree relatives of children with this anomaly.[1]

FEATURES. The foot is dorsiflexed toward the fibular side of the lower leg (Fig. 2–4). This often results in posterior displacement of the lateral malleolus in association with pressure-induced deficiency of subcutaneous adipose tissue at the presumed site of folding compression, and in unusual skin creases at the site of the dorsiflexion of the foot at the ankle (Fig. 2–4). The heel may be in valgus position relative to the ankle, but the bones of the foot itself are usually in normal alignment.

MANAGEMENT, PROGNOSIS, AND COUNSEL. The foot is most commonly flexible. With no therapy or with passive stretching toward a normal position, there is usually a rapid return toward normal form. If the improvement is not rapid, then taping may be utilized. If the situation has not resolved by four to six months, the use of night braces and/or casting merits consideration. The frequency of this deformity by history in first degree relatives (parents and siblings) is 2.6 per cent.[1]

DIFFERENTIAL DIAGNOSIS. The deformity may be secondary to neurological deficiency, as in meningomyelocele.

Congenital vertical talus is a rather rare inherited deformity that may yield a foot in similar position to calcaneovalgus at birth. There is muscle atrophy and the foot is stiff. The calcaneus is displaced posteriorly, and the talus is displaced downward, yielding a rocker-bottom foot. These are difficult to treat and usually require early casting and early surgery to achieve a functional foot.

Reference

1. Wynne-Davies, R.: Family studies and aetiology of club foot. J. Med. Genet. 2:227, 1965.

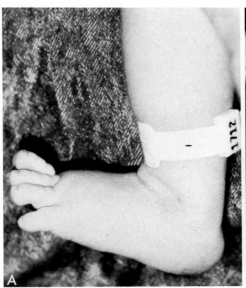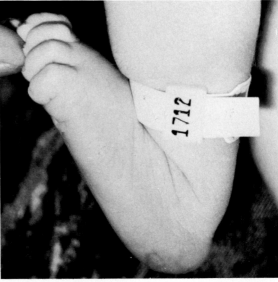

Figure 2–4. *A*, Gentle pressure (right) re-creates the presumed in-utero position of this foot, which engendered the calcaneovalgus positioning.

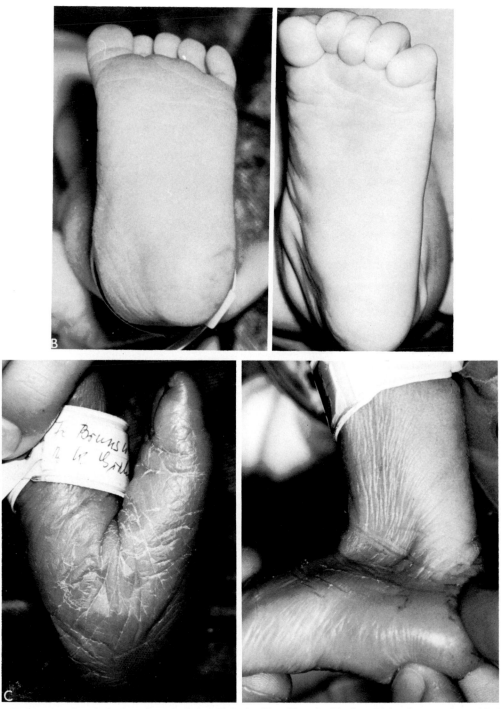

Figure 2–4 *Continued.* *B,* Left, the valgus deviation of the heel is evident in this view. Right, the same foot with simple manipulation at 12 weeks. *C,* Left, medial view of a severely molded calcaneovalgus foot. With ventriflexion of the foot, the lateral view shows the creases, the shallow sulcus, and the posterior displacement of the lateral malleolus and valgus position of the heel, which are the consequences of long-term dorsilateral positioning of the foot in utero.

1.2 Metatarsus Adductus

GENESIS. Compression of the forefoot with the legs flexed across the lower body in late gestation may be one cause of metatarsus adductus, which has a frequency of about 1.2 per 1000 births and an 80 per cent predilection for the male.[1] This may be aggravated by the infant sleeping on the abdomen with the knees tucked up and the lower legs and feet rolled in.

FEATURES. The predominant feature is adduction of the forefoot, often with some supination. The ankle and heel are generally in normal position (Fig. 2–5A).

MANAGEMENT, PROGNOSIS, AND COUNSEL. For mild and flexible cases, manipulative stretch and avoidance of sleeping postures that tend to augment the deformity are all that are usually required. If, after several months, the sleeping posture is tending to augment the deformity, then attempts to change the posture may be of value. In the experience of Dr. Sig. T. Hansen, Jr., at the University of Washington, several devices have been useful.[2] One is putting the child in a heavy sleeper, which keeps the child warm and causes him or her to sprawl rather than tuck in the legs. The leggings of the sleeper may be pinned or sewn together at the knees, making it difficult to achieve the deforming posture. If this is not helpful, a pair of open-toed straight-last shoes with the heels tied together may be placed on the child. If simpler measures fail, reversed-last open-toed shoes tied at the heels may be tried for night-time wear, or the shoes may be connected by a short Denis-Browne or Fillauer splint to provide mild outward rotation (Fig. 2–5). It may be necessary to augment this by early reversed-last shoes in order to maintain the corrected form.

If, when first treated, the foot cannot be passively placed in the neutral position, it is generally wiser to achieve initial correction by very careful casting. If there is associated internal tibial torsion, as frequently happens, a long leg cast is utilized; however, if there is no internal tibial torsion, a short leg cast is usually adequate. The hindfoot and midfoot should be carefully maintained in their neutral positions during the casting. Early management may be critical, since the metatarsus adductus tends to become less flexible with time. The recurrence risk in first degree relatives is 1.8 per cent.[1]

References

1. Wynne-Davies, R.: Family studies and aetiology of club foot. J. Med. Genet. 2:227, 1965.
2. Hansen, S. T.: The child's foot: Evaluation and treatment. Independent Learning Program, School of Medicine, University of Washington, 1978.

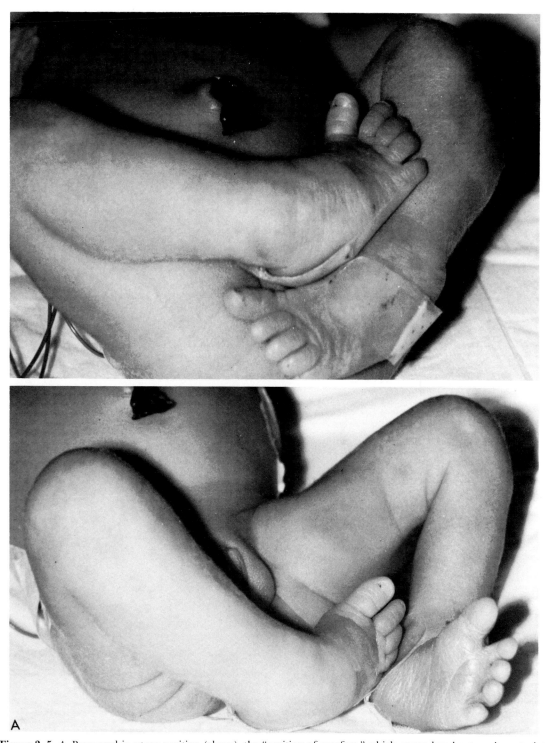

Figure 2–5. *A*, Presumed in-utero position (above), the "position of comfort," which engendered external constraint molding of right forefoot into the metatarsus adductus position shown below.

Illustration continued on following page

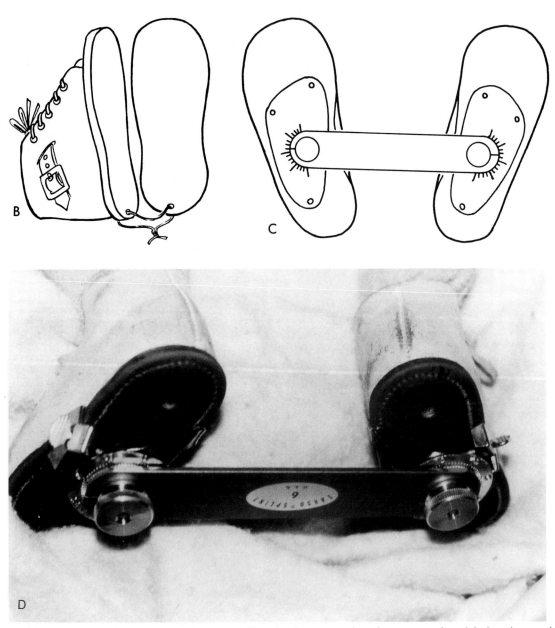

Figure 2–5 *Continued. B,* Simple method for controlling sleeping posture by using open-toed straight-last shoes and tying the heels together with a show laced through holes punched in the heels. *C,* Denis-Browne splint or similar Fillauer bar may be placed on sleeping shoes to prevent deforming sleeping posture. The bar should be relatively short. *D,* Fillauer bar used to correct sleeping posture.

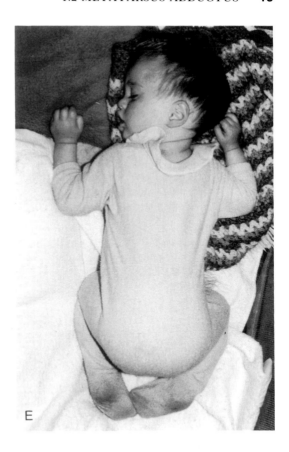

Figure 2–5 *Continued. E,* This infant characteristically slept on his stomach with his knees flexed and his toes turned in. This resulted in bilateral metatarsus adductus. *F,* Management was directed toward trying to correct the sleeping posture by turning the feet out with a Fillauer bar.

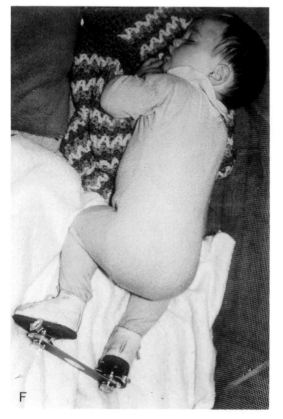

1.3 Equinovarus

("Clubfoot")

GENESIS. This is often a serious foot defect, with up to 50 per cent of cases requiring surgical intervention. Although it is not possible to state with assurance the proportion of equinovarus foot defects that represent constraint foot deformities, it is most likely about one third to one half of cases. The overall frequency is 1.2 per 1000,[1] but this varies among racial groups. For example, in Polynesians the frequency is 12 times higher.[2] The overall sex predilection is 2:1 in favor of the male. However, when the mild "postural equinovarus" cases are considered, there is about a 2:1 propensity toward the female.[1] The most common positional equinovarus deformity is considered to be the result of uterine constraint on the folded legs, especially in the situation of oligohydramnios.

FEATURES. The forefoot is inverted, as are the heel and the whole foot, which is in plantar flexion (Fig. 2–6). There is often a varus deformation of the neck of the talus and a medial shift of the navicular on the head of the talus. The calf muscles may be deficient with shortening. The fibrous capsules of the joints may be thickened on the lateral aspect of the foot. If there has been a long-term compression over the lateral margin of the foot, there may be thin skin with a deficiency of subcutaneous tissue at that site.

MANAGEMENT, PROGNOSIS, AND COUNSEL. Early and rigorous management is merited. If there is flexibility to the foot, initial manipulation and stretch taping toward dorsiflexion of the foot with eversion of the heel should be tried. Maintenance of the corrected position may sometimes need to be fostered by casting and/or Denis-Browne splints in order to prevent a lapse toward the deformed position. If continued improvement does not occur after one to three months of conservative management, or if there is little or no flexibility in the foot (especially the ability to bring the hindfoot equinus into a normal position), then early surgical intervention seems merited. About 40 to 50 per cent of cases arrive at surgery, and about one third of this latter group are improved. If correction is not obtained by one year of age it is unlikely to be fully achieved. The surgery usually involves lengthening of the Achilles tendon, division of the posterior ankle capsule talofibular ligament, and release of the tibialis posterior, flexor hallucis, and digitorum longus if they are unduly tight.

There has not been a clear separation of postural equinovarus and non-constraint-induced equinovarus. From my experience, I believe the prognosis for restoration toward normal form is much better when the cause is uterine constraint in an otherwise normal child. The general recurrence risk of equinovarus defect is 3 per cent.[1] When only the postural equinovarus cases are considered, the recurrence risk is 2.6 per cent.[1]

DIFFERENTIAL DIAGNOSIS. The etiology for the type that is not constraint induced, has a predilection for males, and varies in racial incidence is unknown. It tends to be more rigid than constraint-induced deformation, and there is more likely to be atrophy of calf muscles. The talus tends to be hypoplastic and altered in form. There is even a question whether the primary defect may not be in talonavicular development.

When equinovarus is a feature of neuromuscular disorders, limb deficiency, or a skeletal dysplasia, the prognosis for achieving a normal form to the foot is usually poor. Equinovarus foot deformities may accompany certain neurological deficiencies, especially the spinal cord defect that occurs so frequently with meningomyelocele. An infant with equinovarus defect should be checked for the obvious meningomyelocele and given a close inspection of the lower spine for hemangiomata, hairy nevus, or other subtle clues to an underlying spinal cord defect. A cautious neurological evaluation is also indicated. Partial degrees of equinovarus position occur in a number of cerebral palsy disorders.

Deficiency of the tibia (tibial hemimelia) often results in an equinovarus foot defect. One or more amniotic bands around the leg, proximal to the foot, may result in an equinovarus foot. The defect may be part of an arthrogryposis disorder such as amyoplasia, in which the inward rotation of the hands and shoulders may allow an overall diagnosis (Fig. 2–2). In the amyoplasia form of arthrogryposis, the equinovarus deformity may represent intrinsic deformation due to a primary neuromuscular disorder. Finally, equinovarus may be one feature of a skeletal dysplasia such as diastrophic dwarfism, a syndrome that includes small stature with short limbs, unduly short thumbs, and hypertrophy of ear cartilage (Figs. 1–1 and 2–3). This represents an example of a connective tissue dysplasia that leads to malformation of a joint.

References

1. Wynne-Davies, R.: Family studies and aetiology of club foot. J. Med. Genet. 2:227, 1965.
2. Chung, C. S., Nemechek, R. W., Larson, I. J., and Ching, G. H. S.: Genetic and epidemiological studies of clubfoot in Hawaii. Hum. Hered. *19*:321, 1969.

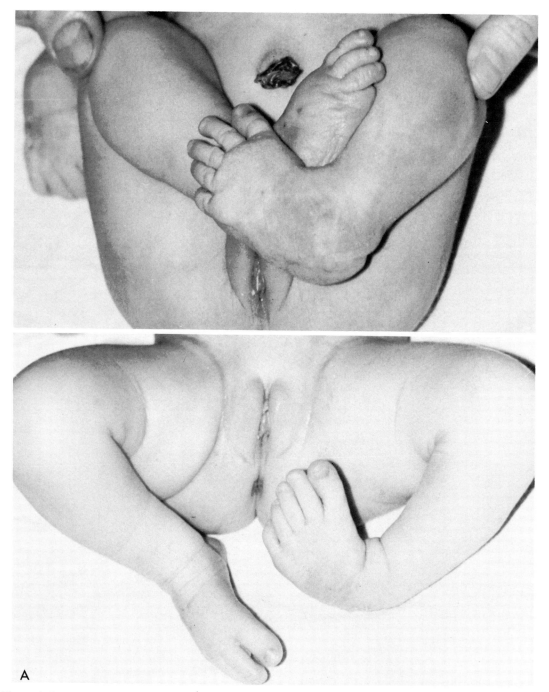

A

Figure 2–6. Equinovarus. *A,* Presumed in-utero position that engendered the equinovarus deformation of the left foot. At the site of in-utero compression over the left lateral ankle the skin is very thin with a fine erythematous reaction, secondary to prolonged pressure.

Illustration continued on following page

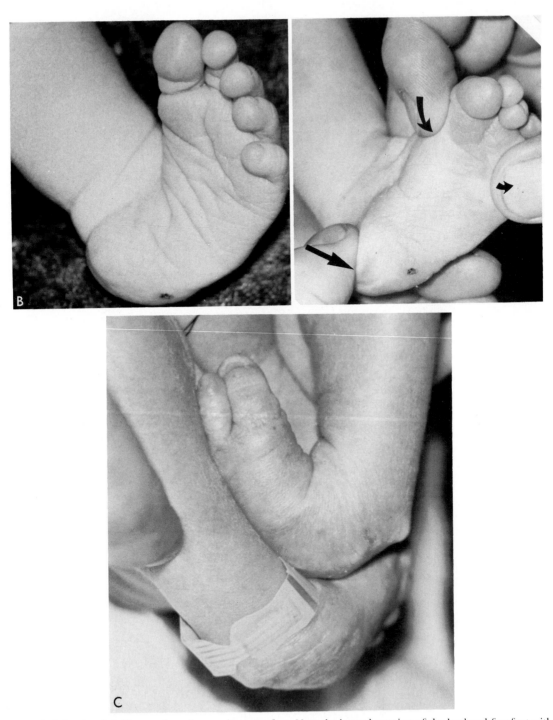

Figure 2–6 *Continued. B,* Plantar view of an equinovarus foot. Note the inward rotation of the heel and forefoot with the whole foot deviated inward at the ankle. Outward pressure on the heel and forefoot resulted in partial correction toward a neutral foot positioning. These feet were corrected by taping and manipulation alone. *C,* Presumed in-utero position that yielded rather severe equinovarus deformation by birth. Note the prominent lateral malleolus over which the skin was very thin.

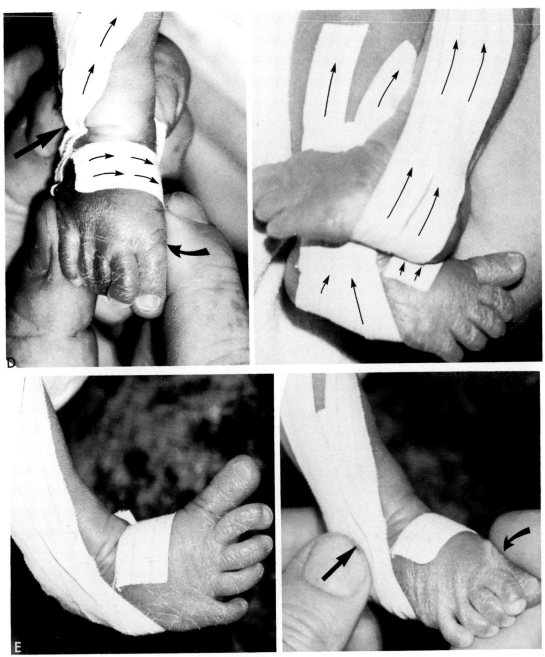

Figure 2–6 *Continued. D,* After manipulating the foot of the patient shown in *C* into a more normal position, several layers of adhesive tape are applied (tincture of benzoin on skin), starting over the dorsum of the foot and bringing the tape medialward under the sole and up the lateral side of the leg. After taping, the feet tend to return partially to their pretaped position, as shown to the right. *E,* When the foot is taped and partially corrected, it is possible for the parents to repeatedly manipulate the foot toward the ideal position, a mode of management that is not possible when the foot is in a cast.

1.4 Deformed Toes

GENESIS. Constraint of the feet while the legs are in a flexed and folded position can result in medial overlapping of the toes, especially the fifth, fourth, and third.

FEATURES. The fifth, fourth, and third toes tend to overlap medially with mild to moderate incurvature (Fig. 2–7). There may be accentuated longitudinal creasing in the sole of the foot where it has been "folded" by external compression.

MANAGEMENT AND PROGNOSIS. If the toes do not readily tend to realign after birth, then manipulative lateral stretching and/or taping is merited. Rarely is later surgery necessary.

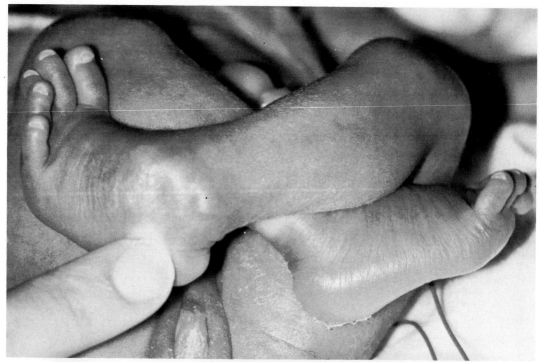

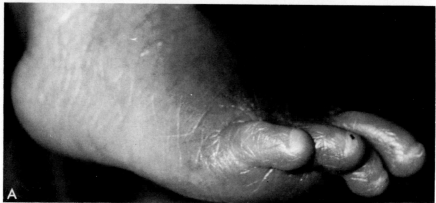

Figure 2–7. Deformed toes. *A*, Presumed position in utero in which uterine constraint compressed the forefeet, resulting in overlapping of the toes.

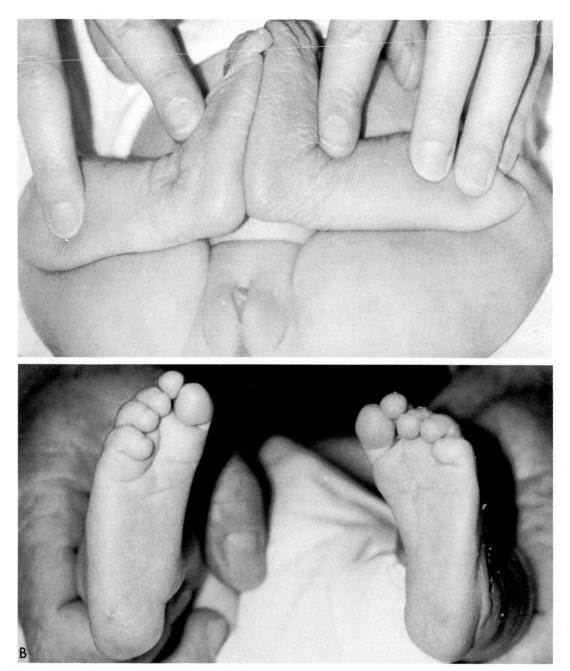

Figure 2–7 *Continued. B,* Presumed positioning in utero in which uterine constraint compressed the feet, yielding unilateral partially folded forefoot and deformation of toes. Note the thin, wrinkled skin over the lateral malleolus (to viewer's left), which is a strong clue that constraint induction of the deformation occurred.

2. TIBIAL TORSION

(Tibial Inbowing)

GENESIS. Torsion of the tibia is sufficiently common in the normal newborn to be considered a normal variant. However, this inbowing occurs to an unusual degree in about 3 per cent of newborns and is especially likely with constraint of the legs in the folded and flexed position. For this apparent reason it is a frequent feature in positional equinovarus deformity, which derives from similar mechanical constraint.

FEATURES. The tibia is medially rotated, with the most acute incurving occurring distally. This tends to angle the plantar surfaces of the feet toward each other. There may also be mild to moderate pes varus in association with medial tibial "torsion."

MANAGEMENT, PROGNOSIS, AND COUNSEL. Seldom is any management required. Following release from the constraint there tends to be progressive straightening of the legs. However, sleeping posture may tend to foster persistence of the tibial torsion. The same preventive measures for sleeping posture as mentioned for metatarsus adductus may be employed. If tibial torsion persists into the second year, night splinting may be indicated (Fig. 2–5D).

DIFFERENTIAL DIAGNOSIS. The lower legs may be more bowed than usual because of a neuromuscular disorder such as meningomyelocele. Problems in bone formation may also result in malleable or fragile bones, such as occur with hypophosphatasia (malleable), osteogenesis imperfecta (fragile), or achondroplasia (tissue dysplasia).

3.0 JOINT DISLOCATION, ESPECIALLY OF HIP

GENERAL. Joints normally develop secondarily within the condensed mesenchyme that will form the bones. Hence a dislocated joint always represents a displacement of the bone from the original site of the joint. Once a joint has been dislocated, it is obvious that the joint capsule has been stretched into an unusual form and that any ligamentous attachment, such as the ligamentum teres of the hip joint, has been elongated and deformed. If the dislocation is of sufficient duration, the aberrant forces will alter the form of the original joint socket. The occurrence of dislocation is dependent on at least three factors, as shown in Figure 2–8A. The joint that is most liable to dislocation is the hip joint because of the major forces that may be brought to bear on it by such situations as breech presentation in later fetal life and because of the sloping angulation of the acetabulum. The second most common dislocation is of the proximal head of the radius, and the third most common dislocation is at the knee, yielding a genu recurvatum. Because of the relative importance and frequency of dislocation of the hip, it will be given more extensive coverage.

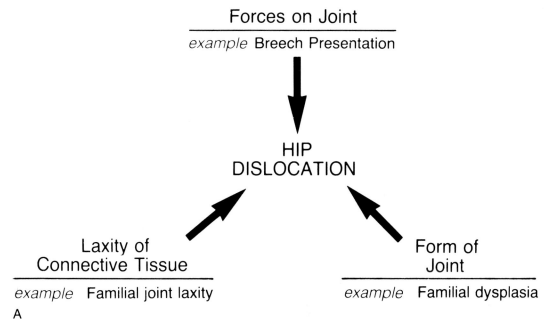

A

Figure 2–8. *A,* Factors that interact in the genesis of joint dislocation with examples that relate to hip dislocation.

Illustration continued on following page

3.1 Hip Dislocation

GENESIS. Figure 2–8 depicts some of the interacting factors that relate to the genesis of hip dislocation. Laxity of connective tissue is an important factor. The 4:1 to 5:1 predilection toward the female is considered to be the consequence of the female fetus being more lax than the male fetus. Arena and Smith[1] suggested that this is the consequence of a lack of testosterone effect in the female fetus. Testosterone, present in the male fetus, results in tougher connective tissue. This has been demonstrated in the hip capsule of the young rodent.[2] Dunn has shown the excess of dislocation of the hip in the female to be as high as 13:1 when it is an isolated deformation.[3] However, when there are multiple deformations, the sex ratio is closer to equality. Carter and Wilkinson found that laxity of three or more joints, noted in 7 per cent of individuals overall, was present in 22 per cent of the first degree relatives of sporadic cases of dislocation of the hip.[4] This suggests a possible heritable tendency toward increased joint laxity. When there were multiple cases of dislocation of the hip in a family, an impressive 65 per cent of first degree relatives had undue joint laxity.[4]

The forces that tend to thrust the head of the femur out of the acetabulum cause a stretching of the joint capsule and of the ligamentum teres (Fig. 2–8C). These forces are most commonly the result of constraint in late fetal life. Since these forces are more likely to affect the first offspring, dislocation of the hip is more common in the first born. Certain presentations during late gestation are particularly likely to cause dislocation of the hip. Breech presentation is notorious in this respect. About 50 per cent of cases of hip dislocation had been breech presentations at birth.[3] In all breech term births (about 3.5 per cent of births) there is a 17 per cent frequency of dislocation of the hip, and for breech with extended legs in utero (frank breech), the incidence is 25 per cent.[3] Breech presentation with the buttocks in the maternal pelvis and the fetal hips tightly flexed upon the abdomen tends to mechanically thrust the femoral heads out of the acetabulum, especially when the legs are extended and "caught" between the abdomen of the fetus and the uterine wall.

The fact that the fetus more commonly lies with its left side toward the mother's spine may be responsible for the increased propensity for the

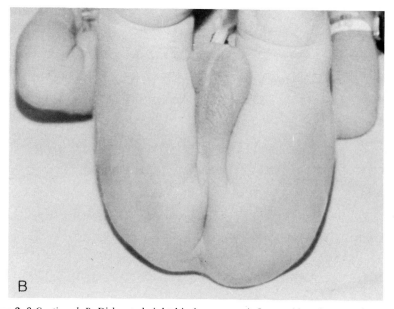

B

Figure 2–8 *Continued. B,* Dislocated right hip in a young infant, evident by gross inspection.

left hip to be dislocated rather than the right.[3] Oligohydramnios, causing overall constraint of the fetus, is associated with an increased frequency of hip dislocation, at least partially the consequence of the increased frequency of breech presentation with oligohydramnios.

The position of the infant *after birth* is also important in the genesis of dislocation of the hip. The hip joint may be lax at birth and only become dislocated postnatally.[5] Undue leg extension in early infancy is considered a factor in the postnatal genesis of hip dislocation.[4] Thus, the hip that has been flexed with a relatively contracted psoas muscle in utero is more likely to be thrust out of its socket by forced extension of the leg. The increased frequency of dislocation of the hip in American Indians and in the Lapps has been at least partially attributed to their practice of swaddling young infants with the legs extended. On the other hand, the relatively low incidence of hip dislocation in the Hong Kong Chinese has been attributed to the mothers' custom of carrying the babies on their lower back with the hips flexed and partially abducted, which mechanically favors maintenance of the femoral head in the acetabulum.

All gradations of dislocation from partially stretched dislocatable hip to fully dislocated hip occur with an overall frequency of about 1 per cent. Considering the full spectrum, Barlow[6] observed that 60 per cent of these dislocatable hips are stable in the normal location by one week of age, and 88 per cent are stable by two months of age. The remaining 12 per cent represent frank dislocation of the hip that was evident at birth or during early infancy, a frequency of 1.2 per 1000.

FEATURES. The usual direction of the dislocation is posterior. The major problem with dislocation of the hip is that it is seldom readily evident on gross inspection of the newly born baby and may not *become* evident until early postnatal life. Thus, diagnosis of congenital hip dislocation involves a cautious physical examination, searching for signs of the whole dislocation spectrum, from a lax dislocatable hip to the dislocated hip that can still be relocated into the acetabulum to the dislocated hip that cannot be relocated. The following type of hip examination is warranted for all newborn babies.

It is of utmost importance that the infant be relaxed during the hip examination. A pacifier or bottle may be of value in this regard. With the infant in the supine position and the hips and knees flexed to 90 degrees and mildly abducted, the examiner, who is facing the baby's buttocks, grasps each thigh. The thumb of each hand is placed on the medial part of the upper thigh and the third finger is placed over the lateral aspect of the upper thigh at the level of the greater trochanter. The first maneuver is to pull out quite gently on the thigh and at the same time push the

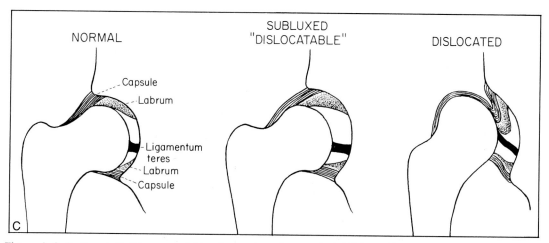

Figure 2–8 *Continued. C,* The normal hip, the moderately stretched "dislocatable" hip, and the overly stretched dislocated hip. (From Clarren, S., and Smith, D. W.: Congenital deformities. Pediatr. Clin. North Am. *24:*665, 1977.)

upper thigh medialward with the third finger. If the hip is dislocated posteriorly—the usual direction for dislocation—and can be relocated, the examiner will feel a noticeable "clunk" as the femoral head slips over the acetabular shelf and into the acetabular socket. If the result of this maneuver is negative, then the second maneuver is to pull out gently on the thigh while at the same time pushing the upper thigh lateralward with the thumb. If this results in a noticeable (palpable) "clunk," as the femoral head is forced over the acetabular rim into a posteriorly dislocated position, the hip may be referred to as dislocatable. (It may also be referred to as an unstable hip.) Minor clicks may be noted in about one third of the examinations and do not appear to be of any consequence. Rather, it is the palpable "clunk" or "thunk" that is relevant.

It is *most* important to appreciate that neither of these above maneuvers will be positive for the hip that is dislocated and cannot be manually relocated. This hip will usually show a limitation in abduction; the greater trochanter may be felt to be posteriorly and superiorly displaced; and the upper leg may appear relatively short. When the dislocation is unilateral or asymmetric in degree, there may be asymmetry in the relative length of the legs, though the lower legs and feet will be the same length. There may also be an obvious discrepancy in the creases of the thigh folds between the two sides. The same type of examination is indicated in the first one or two postnatal examinations after discharge from the newborn nursery. At this time the prior maneuvers, which are routine in the newborn, are of relatively little value. It is paramount to appreciate that not all dislocation of the hip is detected in the newborn nursery and that detectional surveil-

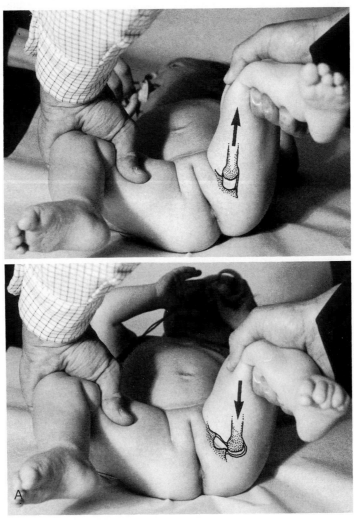

Figure 2–9 *A,* Technique of Barlow maneuver, which assists in detecting the unstable dislocatable hip, which is in the acetabulum. The leg is forcibly pulled up during the upper maneuver. Passage over the rim usually yields a noticeable "clunk." (Courtesy of Dr. Lynn Staheli, University of Washington.)

lance during early infancy is merited.[5] Roentgenograms, which are of little value in the newborn because of the incomplete ossification of the acetabulum and lack of ossification in the femoral head, become more valuable after several months of age to detect evidence of dislocation when clinical suspicion of such a problem exists.

A number of aberrations in morphogenesis may occur as secondary features to dislocation of the hip. They are dependent on the age of development and the duration and extent of the dislocation. These include deformation of the femoral head, imperfect articular cartilage, adherence between the articular surface of the femoral head and the capsular tissue, short psoas, adductor, and hamstring muscles, anteversion at the hip, development of a false acetabulum, and elongation of the ligamentum teres with stretched joint capsule. When such changes are profound, it may be difficult or even impossible to accomplish a closed replacement of the femoral head into its original acetabulum.

MANAGEMENT, PROGNOSIS, AND COUNSEL.

Early and simple conservative management of dislocation of the hip will usually result in a normal hip by the age of walking. If dislocation of the hip is discovered after one year of age, the condition usually requires prolonged, complicated management and results in varying degrees of lifelong disability. Hence early diagnosis, emphasized above, is a key to successful management.

The most common hip diagnosis at birth is the dislocatable or unstable hip. Even though the femoral head is in a normal position at birth, it is considered best to provide prophylactic splinting of the dislocatable hip to prevent the very real possibility of insidious hip dislocation in early infancy. Such splinting is continued until the hip is held firmly in place by its own connective tissue, which had been stretched prior to birth. The aim of the splinting is to maintain the femoral head in the acetabulum with reliable but not excessive constraint. The recommended position is with the hips flexed about 90 degrees and abducted about

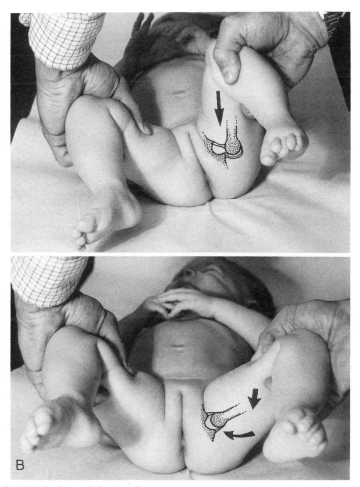

B

Figure 2–9 *Continued. B,* Technique of the Ortolani maneuver, which assists in detecting the dislocated hip, which can be repositioned into the acetabulum. Above, downward pressure further dislocates the hip; below, inward rotation of the hip will force the femoral head over the acetabular rim, leading to a noticeable "clunk." (Courtesy of Dr. Lynn Staheli, University of Washington.)

Illustration continued on following page

25 to 30 degrees. The full frogleg position has been discouraged because the constant, rather excessive forcing of the femoral head into the acetabulum may occasionally result in avascular necrosis in the head of the immobilized femur. There have been a variety of types of splints employed. Probably a pillow splint is not reliable enough. A soft, easily cleaned splint, such as the Plastizote splint, is usually preferable. For the dislocatable hip, a period of four to six weeks of splinting is usually adequate to yield a "tight" hip.

The dislocated hip that can be relocated should be splinted in the above manner, with assurance that the femoral head is staying in the acetabulum. For this hip, the Pavlik splint may be preferable. The duration of splinting varies with the severity of the problem and the age at diagnosis. When detected at birth to one month of age, the mean duration of splinting is 3.6 months, and at one to three months it is seven months. If the dislocation was not detected until three to six months, the mean duration of splinting is 9.3 months.[7]

If it is not possible to reduce the dislocation manually, leg traction should be utilized in an effort to lengthen the contracted muscles and hopefully allow for a closed reduction. If this is not possible, surgical correction is merited. Surgery may include the lengthening or detachment of contracted muscles and reconstruction of the

distorted joint capsule. Surgery is often postponed until the infant is about a year old because of the risk of ischemic necrosis following earlier hip surgery.

Uncorrected dislocation of the hip will adversely affect walking. There is usually a pronounced waddling limp and later development of degenerative hip problems with chronic disability.

The recurrence risk for the more common type of dislocation of the hip is in the range of 3 to 6 per cent, being higher when a boy is affected than when a girl is affected.[4] If both a parent and a child are affected the recurrence risk may be as high as 30 per cent.

DIFFERENTIAL DIAGNOSIS. A malformation problem that itself enhances the likelihood of breech position, or a malformation problem that leads to oligohydramnios (and thereby both excess constraint and enhanced breech positioning), is associated with an increased frequency of dislocation of the hip secondary to the more primary malformation problem.

A number of neurologic disorders may lead to dislocation of the hip, presumably on the basis of diminished muscle strength in holding the femoral head in the acetabulum and/or muscular imbalance. Thus dislocation of the hip may be secondary to meningomyelocele and may occur in certain

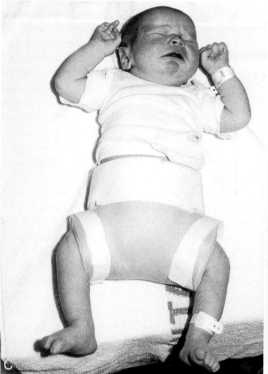 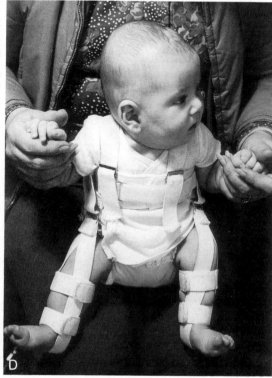

Figure 2–9 *Continued. C,* Plastizote splint utilized for the dislocatable hip in early infancy. *D,* Pavlik splint used for maintaining reposition of the dislocated hip in early infancy.

categories of cerebral palsy, especially when there is flexion and/or adduction spasm at the hip.

In certain types of arthrogryposis (multiple joint contractures) there may be dislocation of the hip. One specific clinical entity in which it occurs is amyoplasia congenita.

Finally, there are a number of syndromes in which dislocation of the hip occurs as a frequent or occasional defect. One of the most striking of these is the Larsen syndrome, in which there tend to be multiple joint dislocations plus an unusually low nasal bridge.

References

General

Lloyd Roberts, G. C.: Orthopaedics in infancy and childhood. New York, Appleton-Century-Crofts, 1971, p. 337.

Staheli, L. T.: Congenital dislocation of the hip. Perinatal Care 2:14, 1978.

Specific

1. Arena, F., and Smith, D. W.: Sex liability to single structural defects. Am. J. Dis. Child. *132*:970, 1978.
2. Hama, H., Yamamuro, T., and Takeda, T.: Experimental studies on connective tissue of the capsular ligament. Acta Orthop. Scand. *47*:473, 1976.
3. Dunn, P. M.: Perinatal observations on the etiology of congenital dislocation of the hip. Clin. Orthop. *119*:11, 1976.
4. Carter, C. O., and Wilkinson, J. A.: Genetic and environmental factors in the etiology of congenital dislocation of the hip. Clin. Orthop. Rel. Res. *33*:March-April, 1964.
5. Place, M., Parkin, P. M., and Fitton, M.: Effectiveness of neonatal screening for congenital dislocation of the hip. Lancet *2*:249, 1978.
6. Barlow, T. G.: Early diagnosis and treatment of congenital dislocation of the hip. J. Bone Joint Surg. *44B*:292, 1962.
7. Hensinger, R. N.: Congenital disloction of the hip. Clin. Symposia *31*:3, 1979.

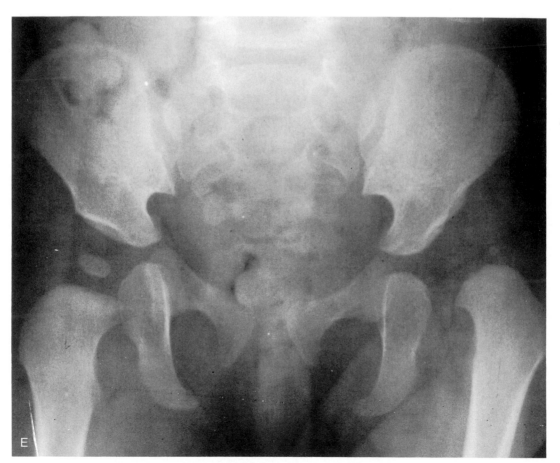

Figure 2–9 *Continued. E,* The secondary changes in acetabulum and neck of femur plus the unseen hour-glass elongation of the hip capsule, elongated ligamentum teres, and foreshortened muscle attachments relating to long-term dislocation of the hip. (Figures are courtesy of Dr. Lynn Staheli, Head of Pediatric Orthopedics, Children's Orthopedic Hospital, Seattle.)

3.2 Knee Dislocation

(Genu Recurvatum)

GENESIS. Hyperextension of the leg with dislocation at the knee most commonly derives from the legs being in extended posture in the breech position. Unusual constraint in a bicornuate uterus and other modes may produce it as well.

FEATURES. There is "backward" curvature of the knee with an unstable and sometimes dislocated knee. The quadriceps muscle tends to be short, and the distal quadriceps may be relatively fibrotic. The patella, a sesamoid bone that normally forms in the quadriceps tendon in response to stress, may be small or absent because of the lack of tension on the quadriceps tendon.

MANAGEMENT, PROGNOSIS, AND COUNSEL. Early adhesive strapping or casting in a corrected position may suffice to bring about a correction by 8 weeks or so in about half of the cases. Recalcitrant cases usually require quadriceps lengthening and sometimes surgical correction of the stretched knee joint capsule and its attachments.

DIFFERENTIAL DIAGNOSIS. Differential diagnosis is similar to that for dislocation of the hip, but knee dislocation is less likely to occur with neurologic disorders and is especially common in the Ehlers-Danlos types of connective tissue disorders (Figs. 2–10 and 2–11).

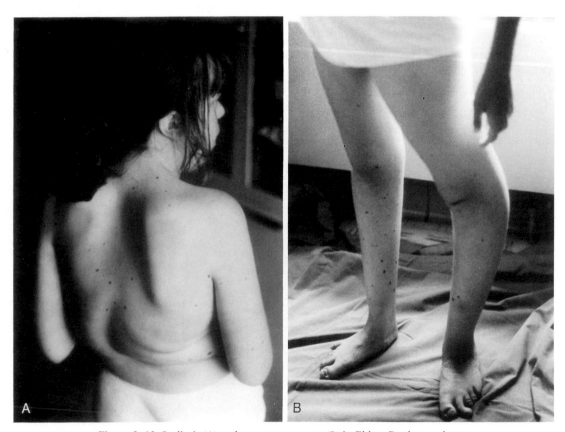

Figure 2–10. Scoliosis *(A)* and genu recurvatum *(B)* in Ehlers-Danlos syndrome.

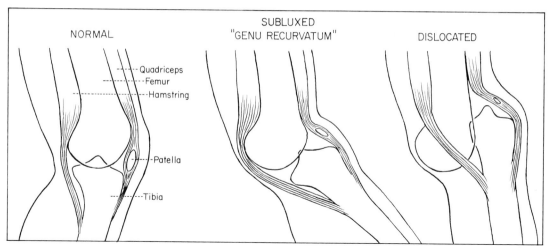

Figure 2–11. Normal knee, stretched tissues to the point of a subluxed "genu recurvatum" (most commonly occurring in prolonged frank breech position) and dislocated knee. The patella develops as a sesamoid bone in the tendon of the quadriceps muscle. With less tension, the sesamoid bone may be small to absent. (From Clarren, S. K., and Smith, D. W.: Congenital deformities. Pediat. Clin. North Am. *24*:665, 1977.)

3.3 Dislocation of the Radial Head

GENERAL. The posterior and lateralward dislocation of the proximal head of the radius, resulting in inability to fully supinate at the elbow, generally gives rise to little disability and is seldom treated. Its genesis is seldom appreciated, although it most commonly occurs in association with dislocation of the hip.

4. NEURAPRAXIAS

(Palsies)

GENESIS. Prolonged compression of a peripheral nerve may lead to palsy, sometimes apparently on the basis of neural ischemia. The frequency of occurrence is about 1.4 per 1000.

FEATURES

Face. Facial nerve palsy is secondary to compression of the facial nerve. Also, ptosis of the eyelid has been observed (Fig. 2–12).

Arm. Radial nerve compression along the humerus due to fetal crowding in late gestation may lead to wrist drop (Fig. 2–13) as a function of radial nerve palsy.[1, 2] Wrist drop may also result from compression of the posterior interosseous nerve, when prolonged intrauterine palmar flexion results in traction on the posterior interosseous nerve over a fixed point at the origin of the nerve in the supinator muscle.[2]

Leg. Sciatic compression may cause weakness in one or both legs. In babies with prolonged breech presentation and extended legs, traction on the sciatic nerve may exert a selective effect on the lateral (external) popliteal nerve due to relative fixation of the nerve at the neck of the fibula. This results in foot drop.[2] Prolonged extreme abduction, flexion, and external rotation of the leg at the hip can result in traction on the obturator nerve as it is stretched between fixation points at the pubic ramus and knee joint. This results in limitation of active internal rotation and adduction of the thigh and in limitation of knee extension.[2, 3]

MANAGEMENT AND PROGNOSIS. There is usually little need for management. When the nerve compression has occurred in late gestation there is usually a full return of function within a matter of days to weeks. If the nerve compression has occurred in early fetal life the consequences are more likely to be permanent, as delineated in 20. Extrauterine Pregnancy.

References

1. Feldman, G. V.: Radial nerve palsies in the newborn. Arch. Dis. Child. 32:469, 1957.
2. Craig, W. S., and Clark, J. M. P.: Of peripheral nerve palsies in the newly born. J. Obstet. Gynaecol. (Brit. Emp.) 65:229, 1958.
3. Craig, W. S., and Clark, J. M. P.: Obturator palsy in the newly born. Arch. Dis. Child. 37:661, 1962.

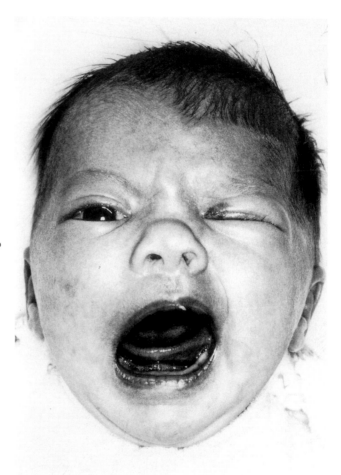

Figure 2–12. Facial nerve palsy leading to ptosis of the eyelid.

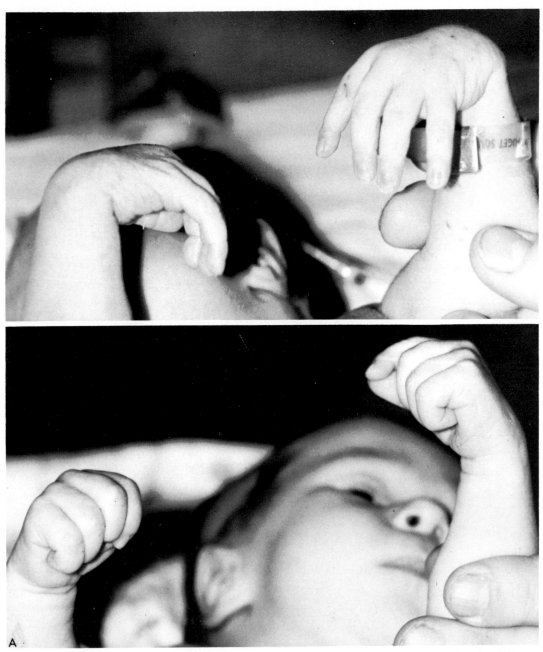

Figure 2–13. *A,* Top, Maximum extension of hands at birth. Radial palsy secondary to constraint of radial nerve between the humerus and the rib cage. Bottom, Same infant at two months of age showing vast improvement in ability to extend the hand at the wrist and to clench the hand.

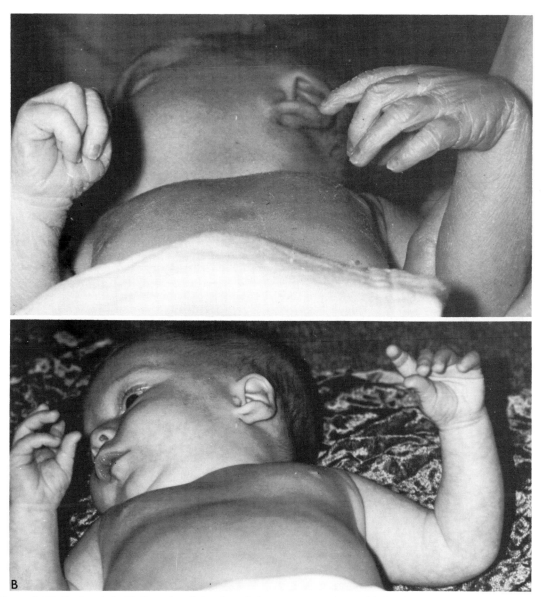

Figure 2–13 *Continued. B,* Unilateral radial palsy relating to compression at birth (above) and 12 weeks later, by which time function was normal. The compression in this instance related to engagement five weeks prior to delivery in a restricted birth canal.

5.0 THORACIC CAGE AND SPINE

5.1 Lung Hypoplasia

GENESIS. Constraint of thoracic cage expansion by such causes as oligohydramnios or small uterine cavity gives rise to this condition.

FEATURES. Pulmonary hypoplasia with limited alveolar development leads to respiratory insufficiency (Fig. 2–14).

MANAGEMENT AND PROGNOSIS. When the thoracic compression has been the result of chronic leakage of amniotic fluid or a small uterine cavity, every measure toward oxygenation should be taken in the hope of maintaining survival until lung development becomes adequate for normal respiration.

DIFFERENTIAL DIAGNOSIS. Oligohydramnios may be the result of inadequate urine flow into the amniotic space, in which case the prognosis is usually grim.

Diaphragmatic hernia not only limits lung development on the side of the hernia but also shifts the mediastinal contents toward the opposite side, thereby limiting lung growth on that side as well.

Hence infants with this condition usually expire of respiratory insufficiency due to lung hypoplasia.

Several skeletal dysplasias have a profound impact on thoracic cage growth and thereby result in respiratory insufficiency. One is thanatophoric dwarfism. The word *thanatophoric* means "death dealing," and death in this condition is usually the consequence of respiratory insufficiency. In a study of chondrodystrophic cho/cho mouse fetuses with pulmonary hypoplasia and restricted thoracic growth due to defective endochondral bone formation, Hepworth, Carey, and Seegmiller demonstrated that decreased thoracic volume prevented normal alveolarization and growth of the fetal lung in late gestation.[1]

Reference

1. Hepworth, W. B., Carey, J. C., and Seegmiller, R. E.: Pathogenesis of pulmonary hypoplasia in mice. Teratology *35*:47A, 1987.

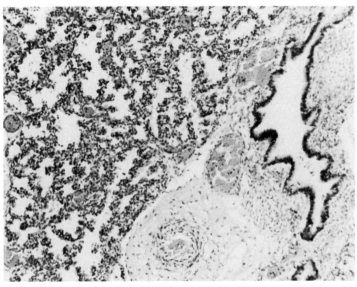

Figure 2–14. Lung hypoplasia in an infant with oligohydramnios. The lung is not adequately developed to allow for respiration.

5.2 Pectus Carinatum or Excavatum

GENESIS. Compression can alter the shape of the thoracic cage and result in depression or protrusion of the sternum (Fig. 2–15).

FEATURES. Pectus excavatum (inward sternum), pectus carinatum (prominent sternum).

MANAGEMENT AND PROGNOSIS. In mild to moderately severe cases no management is usually utilized, and the thoracic cage tends to improve with time. Surgical intervention merits considera-

tion in severe cases for cosmetic reasons; it is unusual for such a deformity to affect respiration.

DIFFERENTIAL DIAGNOSIS. Thoracic deformities may occur concomitantly with abdominal muscle weakness, with a number of neurologic disorders, with some genetic connective tissue disorders, and with a number of recognized syndromes.

A short chorda tendineae of the diaphragm may cause a pectus excavatum, as may prolonged partial airway obstruction with inspiratory stridor.

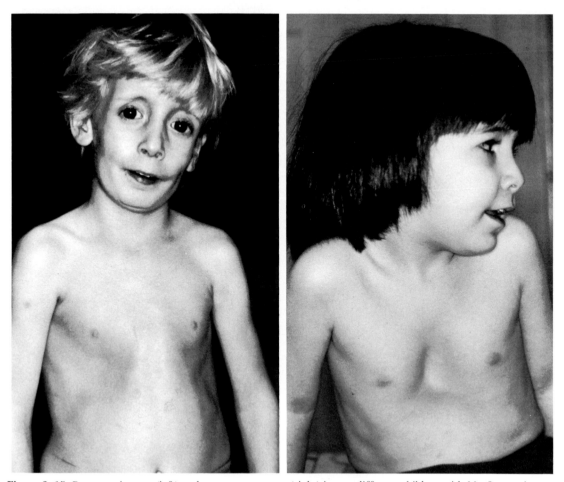

Figure 2–15. Pectus carinatum (left) and pectus excavatum (right) in two different children with Marfan syndrome, an autosomal dominant connective tissue disorder that results in laxity of connective tissues.

5.3 Scoliosis

GENESIS AND FEATURES. External constraint may cause scoliosis. To do so during late gestation, a fairly profound restraint, such as occurs in a transverse lie, is necessary.

MANAGEMENT AND PROGNOSIS. Initial observation with manipulative stretching is merited in order to determine whether or not full reformation will occur after release from the presumed constraint. If there is no progressive improvement, successive bivalve plastic jackets should be made that tend to overcorrect the scoliotic bend.

DIFFERENTIAL DIAGNOSIS. Vertebral anomalies can result in scoliosis, as can neurologic problems that alter muscle tone. Some skeletal dysplasias and connective tissue disorders lead to scoliosis (Figs. 2–12A and 2–16).

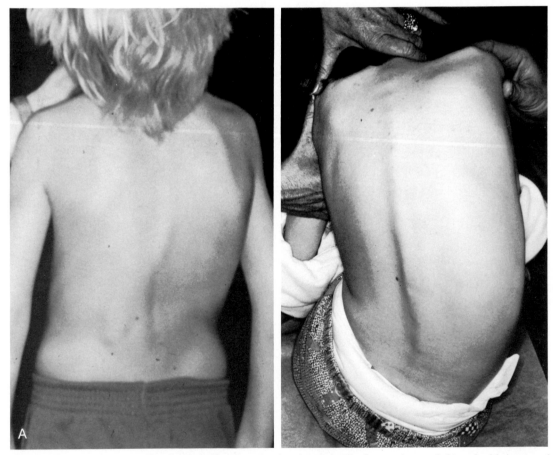

Figure 2–16. *A,* Scoliosis associated with laxity of connective tissues in Marfan syndrome (left) and with increased muscle tone in a young woman with Rett syndrome (right).

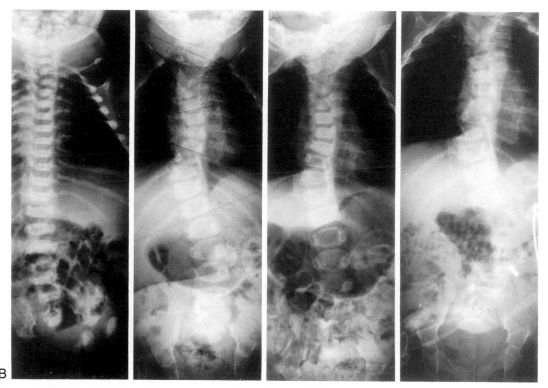

B

Figure 2–16 *Continued. B*, Progressive scoliosis in diastrophic dysplasia, an autosomal recessive skeletal dysplasia that results in abnormal connective tissues. These changes in spinal curvature occurred over the course of the first 18 months of life.

6. NOSE DEFORMATION

GENESIS AND FEATURES. Small nose may result from compressive limitation of nasal growth in face presentation and is often associated with transverse lie and with a small uterine cavity.

Compressed, downcurved nose is a feature of oligohydramnios and severe crowding, such as can occur in a bicornuate uterus (Fig. 2–17).

Deviated nose is not rare and appears to be secondary to external constraint. The lower edge of the nasal cartilage may be dislocated from its placement on the vomerine ridge. This will result in an asymmetric nose with slanting of the columella and a smaller nasal aperture on the side toward which the cartilaginous septum is dislocated. About 2 per cent of newborn babies have an anterior dislocation of the nasal septum, and about 17 per cent have some septum deformation (Fig. 2–18).[1]

MANAGEMENT AND PROGNOSIS. The first two categories generally resolve spontaneously. The dislocated nasal septum should be treated about the third day after birth by repositioning the septal cartilage into the anatomic groove in the floor of the nose. The cartilaginous part of the nose is simply grasped between the thumb and forefinger, using gauze, and lifted forward while a probe or elevator is inserted into the nares below the free edge of the dislocated septum, forcing it into its normal location.[2] A slight nasal asymmetry may persist for several weeks after relocation before the normal form is fully re-established. For the deformed septum that is not dislocated there is no known contraindication to manipulation to reposition the nose in an effort to restore the nasal septum to a normal alignment.

DIFFERENTIAL DIAGNOSIS. Small nose may be a feature in a number of specific disorders.

References

1. Gray, L. P.: Septal and associated cranial birth deformities. Med. J. Aust. *1*:557, 1974.
2. Stoksted, P., and Schønsted-Madsen, U.: Traumatology of the newborn's nose. Rhinology *17*:77, 1979.

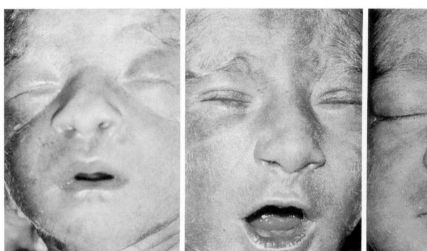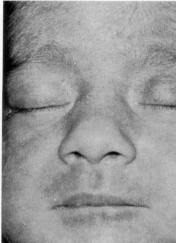

Figure 2–17. Nasal deformation, as can occur with oligohydramnios and severe crowding.

Figure 2–18. *A,* Nasal deviation due to constraint in utero and during delivery. *B,* Top, Deviated nasal septum vs. normal. Middle, The compression test is positive when there has been dislocation of the lower edge of the nasal cartilage (left). The nasal cartilage is unable to return to its former slot in the vomerine ridge. The normal response to compression is shown to the right. Bottom, After reduction of the dislocation of the cartilaginous septum there is still slight asymmetry (left) but the compression test (right) shows that the cartilage is relocated into its slot in the vomerine ridge. (Courtesy of Stoksted, P., and Schønsted-Madsen, U.: Traumatology of the newborn's nose. Rhinology *17*:79, 1979.)

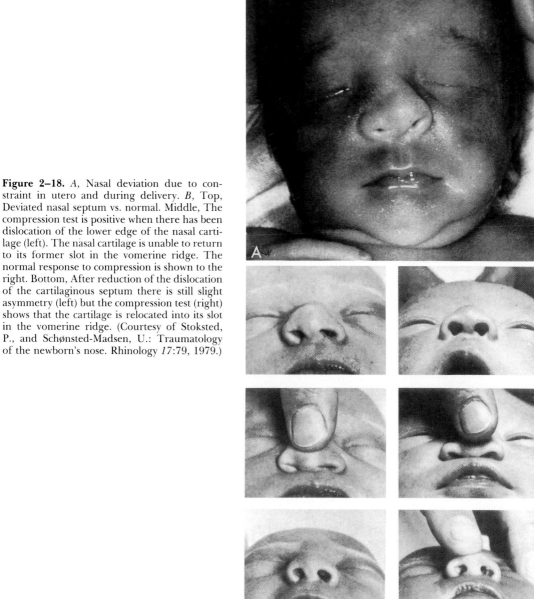

7. EXTERNAL EARS

GENESIS AND FEATURES. *Accordion-type overfolding* of the upper helix and of other parts of the cartilaginous auricle is a frequent constraint deformity, as in *flattening of the ear against the head* (Fig. 2–19).

Appearance of a *low-set ear* may be engendered by molded skewing of the craniofacies, such as can occur with oligohydramnios or the constraint of a bicornuate uterus.

Finally, prolonged constraint of the external ear may result in *asymmetric overgrowth* of the ear.[1]

MANAGEMENT AND PROGNOSIS. Return to normal form within the first few postnatal weeks tends to confirm the deformational origin of such ear defects, which generally require no management.

When the ear is abnormally crumpled into a form that is unlikely to resolve with time, dental wax molds can be individually fashioned and taped in place (Fig. 2–20). This is most effective if done in the first few days of life while the ear cartilage is still relatively soft and pliable.[2]

DIFFERENTIAL DIAGNOSIS. Aberrations of ear form caused by defects in development and/or function of auricular ear muscles, such as protruding auricle and lop ear, do not improve postnatally. A truly low-set ear is a very rare malformation.

References

1. Aase, J. M.: Structural defects as a consequence of late intrauterine constraint: Craniotabes, loose skin, and asymmetric ear size. Sem. Perinatol. 7:270, 1983.
2. Brown, F. E., Colen, L. B., Addante, R. R., and Graham, J. M., Jr.: Correction of congenital auricular deformities by splinting in the neonatal period. Pediatrics 78:406, 1986.

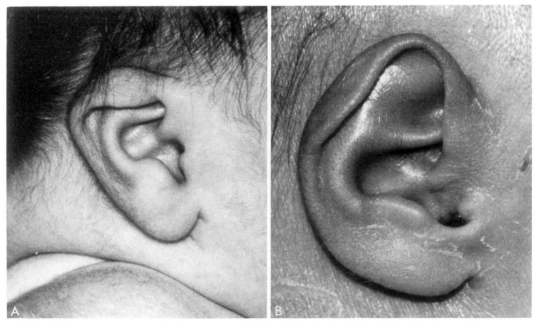

Figure 2–19. *A,* Constraint overfolding of scapha helix. *B,* Partial "crumpling" of ear form, especially concha.

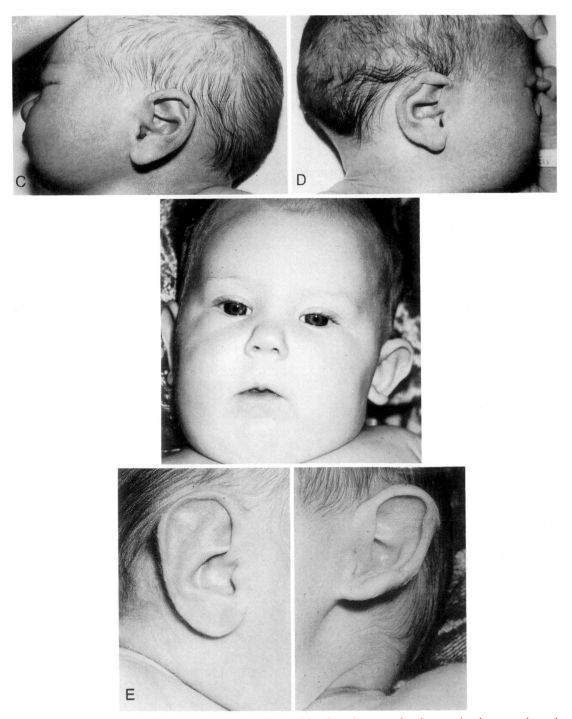

Figure 2–19 *Continued.* C and D, Crumpling of the helix resulting from late gestational constraint due to prolonged oligohydramnios. *E,* Uplifted crumpled ear caused by oblique skewed head position in utero, with the left auricle being caught between the shoulder and head and the right ear relatively flattened against the calvarium. Note the asymmetrical overgrowth of the more compressed right ear.

Illustration continued on following page

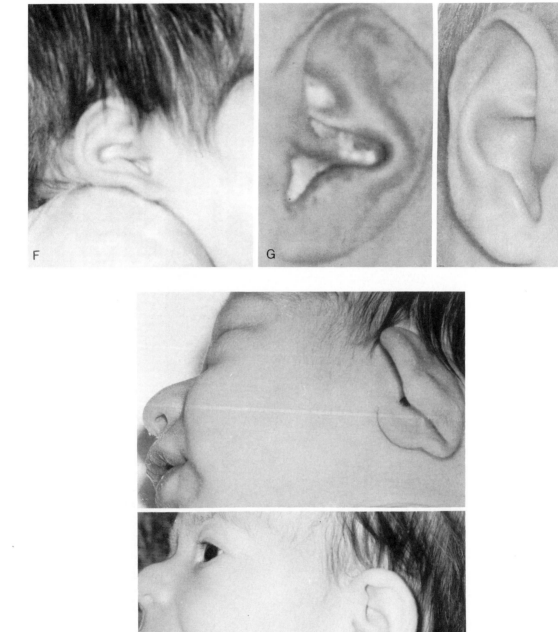

Figure 2–19 *Continued. F,* Uplifted auricle caused by shoulder constraint under auricle in utero. *G,* Auricle flattened against head by oligohydramnios constraint at birth (left) and two months after being relieved from constraint (right). *H,* Top, Folded-over auricle secondary to constraint in an asymmetrical breech presentation in a septate uterus. Bottom, Twelve weeks later the auricle has largely returned to normal form. Taping the ear may accelerate the process of reformation.

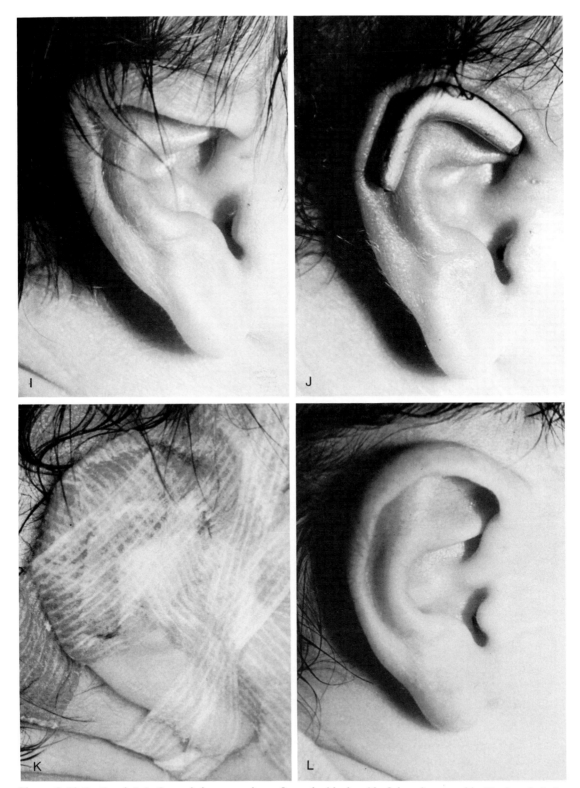

Figure 2–19 *Continued. I–L,* Crumpled ears can be re-formed with the aid of dental wax molds. Moving clockwise from upper left *I* to *L* show the initial form of an ear deformity (I) that required surgery in the infant's mother. Dental wax molds were applied to reshape the ear (J), and these were taped securely in place (K). The ear form remained normal (L) after removal of taping and wax molds.

8. MANDIBLE DEFORMATION

GENESIS AND FEATURES. *Micrognathia* may be caused by the chin being compressed against the chest. If the compression is of prolonged duration there may be a pressure indentation on the upper thoracic surface. Another cause is face presentation, with the mandible being a presenting part (Fig. 2–20).

Mandibular asymmetry with a laterally tilted mandible is most commonly the result of the shoulder having been thrust up under the mandible in a breech presentation or in a prolonged vertex presentation.

MANAGEMENT AND PROGNOSIS. No management is usually required. Postnatally there is usually catch-up growth back to expected mandibular size and form.

DIFFERENTIAL DIAGNOSIS. There are a number of disorders in which micrognathia may be a feature. Asymmetric mandible may occur with hemifacial microsomia.

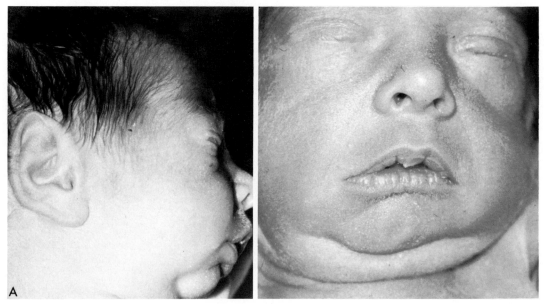

Figure 2–20. *A*, Micrognathia due to constraint. Note the redundancy of skin secondary to constraint-induced overgrowth of skin in the region.

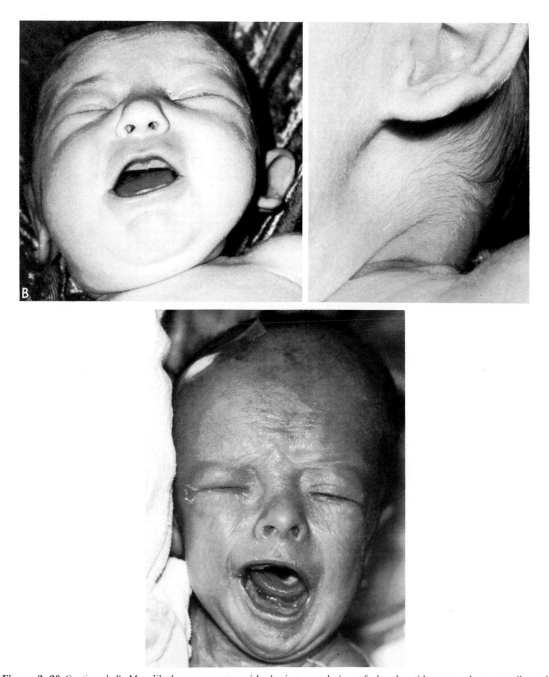

Figure 2–20 *Continued. B,* Mandibular asymmetry with sloping angulation of alveolar ridge secondary to unilateral shoulder compression. Note the sulcus impression made by the shoulder (right). Another infant (bottom) had marked asymmetry secondary to unilateral shoulder compression in utero.

Illustration continued on following page

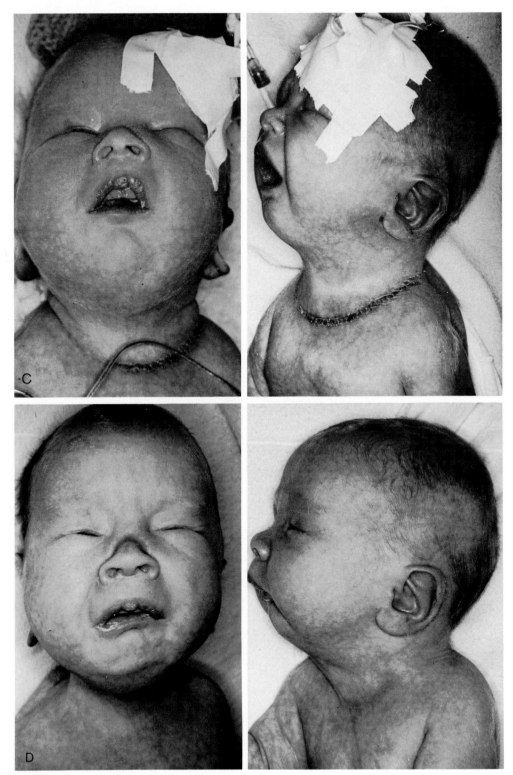

Figure 2–20 *Continued. C,* Marked facial compression with jaw asymmetry and necrosis along anterior neck creases due to prolonged transverse lie with oligohydramnios due to slow leakage of amniotic fluid since the seventeenth week of gestation. Note that by 2 weeks of age *(D),* the necrotic neck folds had healed with scarring, but residual facial asymmetry was present.

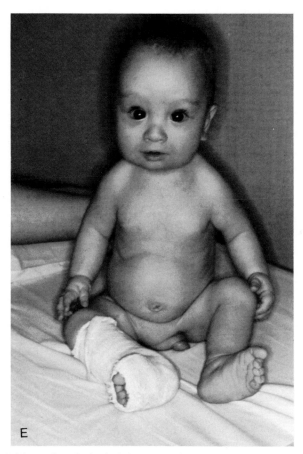

Figure 2–20 *Continued. E*, With continued physical therapy and orthopedic management, there was further return to normal form during the second half of the first year of life.

9. STERNOCLEIDOMASTOID TORTICOLLIS

GENESIS AND FEATURES. Prenatally acquired torticollis usually occurs in conjunction with the rhomboid-shaped (plagiocephalic) head in response to the head being caught askew (Fig. 2–21). These conditions occur together once in every 300 live births.[1] One hypothesis is that the constraint on the side of the neck causes ischemic changes in the middle portion of the sternocleidomastoid muscle, with secondary fibrosis and sometimes a palpable fusiform fibrous mass, the sternocleidomastoid "tumor." The shortening of the musles tends to maintain the aberrant posture of the head and face, the head being tilted toward the affected side, and the chin being rotated toward the opposite, unaffected convex side, the "side facing the sun."[2] Intrauterine constraint accounts for most cases of torticollis and plagiocephaly, and the rhomboid head shape may progress in severity if the infant's head remains turned toward one side postnatally. Eventually, uncorrected torticollis can result in significant facial asymmetry, to such a degree that the eyes are at different levels.

MANAGEMENT AND PROGNOSIS. Mild degrees of torticollis improve spontaneously, especially those without a palpable fusiform fibrous tumor. Neck-stretching exercises and physical therapy are recommended. More rigorous modes of management are set forth under 10. Oblique Head Deformation—Plagiocephaly-Torticollis Sequence. Early diagnosis and management are extremely important, and the presence of a unilateral epicanthal fold or significant asymmetry in the size of the ears (greater than 4 mm difference in size), or both, may be early clues that significant cranial deformation is occurring.[3]

DIFFERENTIAL DIAGNOSIS. Disruptive tearing of the sternocleidomastoid muscle may occur at birth, especially during delivery of the aftercoming head in a vaginal breech delivery.

References

1. Dunn, P. M.: Congenital sternomastoid torticollis: An intrauterine postural deformity. Arch. Dis. Child. *49*:824, 1974.
2. Clark, R. N.: Diagnosis and management of torticollis. Pediat. Ann. *5*:43, 1976.
3. Jones, M. C.: Unilateral epicanthal fold: Diagnostic significance. J. Pediatr. *108*:702, 1986.

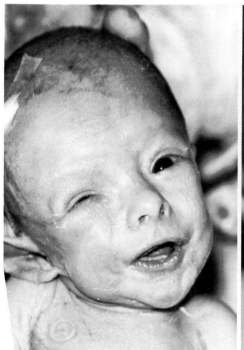 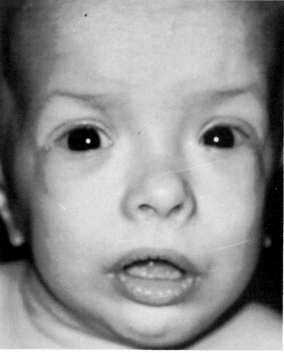

A

Figure 2–21. *A*, Torticollis with shortening of the right sternocleidomastoid muscle as part of the impact of the head being compressed askew onto the right shoulder (left). With conservative stretching, the face was almost symmetrical by several months of age (right).

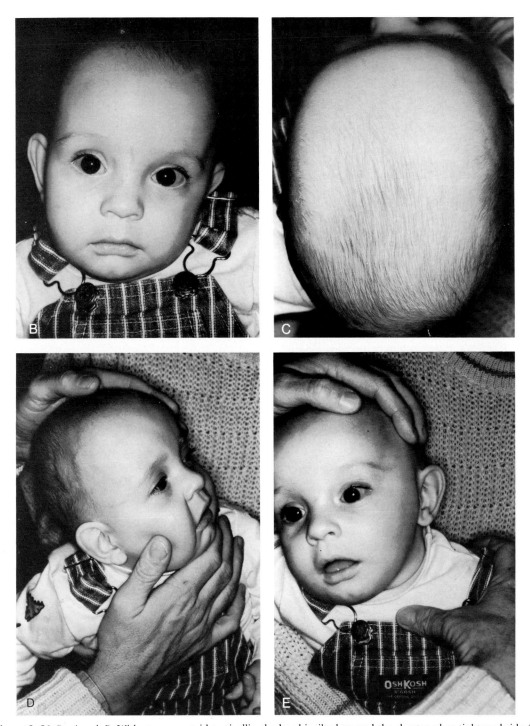

Figure 2–21 *Continued. B*, With sternomastoid torticollis, the head is tilted toward the shortened or tightened side (in this case the left side) and rotated toward the other side. *C*, As the infant rests on his occiput asymmetrically, the right occiput is flattened with advancement of the ear and frontal region on the right. *D*, In order to restore sternomastoid symmetry and prevent progressive plagiocephaly, neck stretching exercises should be done at least five times daily. For left torticollis, gently turn the head to the left side and try to get the chin slightly past the shoulder. *E*, For the neck stretch, place your right hand on the baby's left shoulder and your other hand on the left side of the baby's head. Gently stretch the right ear to the right shoulder. Hold each stretch for at least 20 seconds. (Neck stretching exercises courtesy Pamela J. Valentine, M.C.S.P. & M.C.P.A., Director of Paediatric Physiotherapy, Thames Valley Children's Centre and War Memorial Children's Hospital, London, Ontario, Canada.)

10. OBLIQUE HEAD DEFORMATION— PLAGIOCEPHALY-TORTICOLLIS SEQUENCE

GENESIS. During late fetal life the head may become compressed toward one side (Fig. 2–22). Such obliquity of forces usually results in asymmetric molding of the craniofacies. The same compression may have an adverse effect on the sternocleidomastoid muscle, resulting in ischemic changes in the middle portion of the muscle with or without consequent fibrosis and torticollis. Lopsided head constraint is most likely to occur in first-born babies and in larger babies. The deformations are more commonly left-sided, possibly on the same proposed basis as that for the left-sided predilection for dislocation of the hip: namely, the propensity of the fetus to lie with its left side toward the mother's back.

Plagiocephaly and torticollis occur together once in every 300 live births.[1] Early diagnosis and treatment are important to prevent permanent cosmetic deformity.[2, 3]

FEATURES

Craniofacial and Neck. Oblique molding of the head yields asymmetric prominence of the side of the forehead that is tilted downward, with contralateral prominence of the occiput. The degree of craniofacial distortion may be sufficient to cause a variant placement of the eyes. Major asymmetry of the vertex is most obvious when the head is viewed from above but may be easily missed when the infant is examined face to face. The presence of a unilateral epicanthal fold, usually ipsilateral to the side of occipital flatness, should prompt further investigation for the plagiocephaly-torticollis deformation sequence.[4] The external ear on the compressed side has often been partially folded or thrust out by the compression of the shoulder. It may also be significantly larger, as a manifestation of prolonged compression, than the ear on the noncompressed side.[5] The mandible is often asymmetric and tilted. Scoliosis may be present, as may other deformities such as dislocation of the hips and talipes.[1] The position of comfort is with the head tilted to one side and the neck in the torticollis position. If there has been damage to the sternocleidomastoid muscle on the side that was held askew, this situation may tend to perpetuate the torticollis positioning. Persistent fetal neck rotation may predispose toward venous occlusion in the

contralateral sternocleidomastoid muscle, leading to fibrosis and hence a shorter muscle on that side, resulting in congenital muscular torticollis.[1, 3, 6–8] The asymmetric cranium and neck foster a tendency for the infant to lie on one side of the head or face, in the position of comfort, thus maintaining the deformity.

MANAGEMENT, PROGNOSIS AND COUNSEL. In most instances of plagiocephaly with torticollis, it would seem reasonable to observe the infant during the first two to three months after birth in order to determine whether spontaneous resolution will take place. During this conservative period of observation there are a few procedures that might be worth utilizing. The surface upon which the baby's head rests should be relatively soft, the infant's crib should be placed so that attractive objects such as people and mobiles are on the same side as the torticollis, and the head and neck may be moderately overstretched away from the torticollis several times a day.

With mild to moderate torticollis, early persistence with neck stretching exercises will usually correct the problem and prevent the postnatal plagiocephaly that results from always resting on the same area of the cranium. Usually, the head tilts to one side, and the face turns to the opposite side. For example, with a left torticollis, the head tilts to the left, and the face turns to the right (Fig. 2–22B). To correct this posture, the head should be stretched to the right, so that the right ear is gradually brought to the right shoulder and held there for 20 seconds. Then the head should be turned toward the left so that the chin is brought past the left shoulder and held there for 20 to 60 seconds. For the head stretch to be effective, as the parent faces the baby, the left hand should be on the left side of the baby's face, and the right hand should be on the baby's shoulder, *where it bears down firmly on the shoulder during the stretch.* To correct torticollis appropriately, both exercises must be done together and regularly (at least 5 times each day). After a meal or diaper change is usually a good time to make these exercises a regular part of the daily routine. It is particularly important to initiate early neck and head stretching exercise with severe torticollis.

Another measure that can be utilized is to place a silk or nylon stocking of the proper size to fit snugly, but not tightly, over the baby's calvarium.

The lower part of the stocking is tied into a knot, and the stocking is cut and fitted in such a manner that the knot tends to force the baby to lie on the more prominent side and thus avoid perpetuating the deformity. Care must be taken to avoid suffocating or strangling the infant with this method. It may be simpler to attempt repositioning with carefully placed pillows. If little or no improvement has occurred by two to three months of age, a more rigorous form of management should be considered.

One relatively conservative mode of management is the construction of a Clarren Orthocephalic Helmet, which will restrain growth at the prominent parts of the head but allow the shallow parts of the head to grow.[2, 3] Thus the prominent parts are restrained while brain growth provides the mechanical forces from within the calvarium to round out the shallow or flattened regions. The method begins by making a plaster cast of the infant's deformed head with rapidly drying plaster splint material. By utilizing a stockinette cap, the plaster cast can be readily removed while maintaining its shape. The cast is then inverted and filled with plaster of Paris, into which a one-inch pipe is inserted, so that the completed bust can be mounted on a base for further work. After removing the cast material, plaster of Paris is then

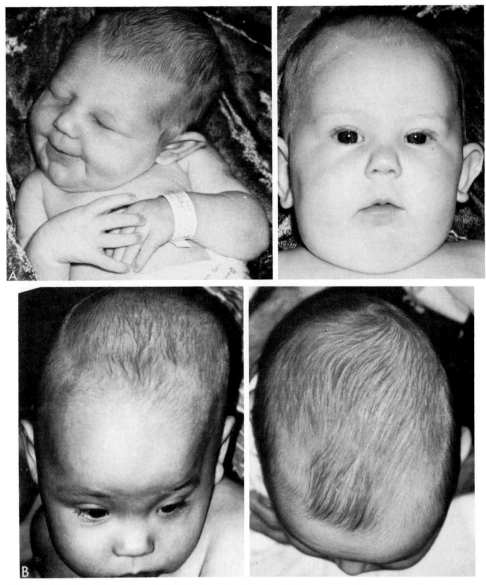

Figure 2–22. *A*, Left, "position of comfort" of a large baby who had been in an oblique presentation for some weeks before delivery, yielding the lopsided head with torticollis. Right, same baby at five months of age showing marked improvement from manipulation alone. The auricle, though improved, is still moderately deformed. *B*, Varying degrees of oblique-shaped plagiocephalic heads in two young infants.

added to the model where the head is shallow, but none is added where the head is unduly prominent. Thus a more ideally shaped head is modeled. From the new model, a plastic helmet is made, much like an American football helmet. It is tight where the infant's head is prominent and allows for growth in the less prominent regions. Once brain growth has filled out the helmet, no further management is usually needed. If there is accompanying muscular torticollis, it is important to institute active and passive neck-stretching exercises to restore neck muscle symmetry. If helmet therapy is utilized by two to four months of age, it usually requires only two to three months to re-form the head to a more normal shape. However, if the helmet management is not employed until seven to eight months of age, it may require four to five months to achieve the desired result. The pace of re-formation relates to the rate of brain growth, which is much more rapid during the first six months than later in infancy.

Other modes of management that have been utilized include resection of the sternocleidomastoid muscle. This may be considered in the second or third year if the foregoing measures have not been successful. Hopefully the more conservative Clarren Orthocephalic Helmet and vigorous neck physical therapy will obviate the need for this procedure.

The majority of mild to moderately severe instances of plagiocephaly with torticollis improve to normal with just neck physical therapy, but most instances of severe plagiocephaly-torticollis deformation sequence will require helmet therapy the achieve complete resolution.[9] The practice of artificial postnatal head deformation is an ancient one practiced by many earlier cultures.[9, 10]

DIFFERENTIAL DIAGNOSIS. A malformation of the cervical vertebrae may be the primary cause of the head being askew, in which case the deformation of plagiocephaly and torticollis would be secondary to an intrinsic malformation problem. In such relatively rare instances, it may be necessary to use more than one helmet to achieve the desired cranial symmetry (Fig. 2–23).

A neuromuscular disorder may be the primary cause of the head being askew; in such instances, prolonged helmet therapy may also be required.

Asymmetric craniostenosis of coronal or lambdoidal sutures may produce an asymmetric head. However, it is usually possible to distinguish constraint deformation from craniostenosis by the prenatal history, clinical appearance, palpation of the suture lines, and the natural history after birth—without utilizing roentgenography or other studies. (See subsequent section.)

Postnatally, neuromuscular disorders, particularly those predisposing toward hypotonia, and occasionally severe neglect, may cause an infant to lie in a particular position for a prolonged period of time, long enough to give rise to asymmetric molding of the head. This can usually be distinguished from congenital constraint plagiocephaly by the history at birth and the natural history after birth. Prolonged positioning in a straight-backed infant seat can result in marked occipital flattening, similar to that seen with purposeful cranial deformation by various primitive cultures (Fig. 2–24).

Prematurely born infants usually have poor muscle tone and relatively malleable heads. If they persistently lie on a firm surface toward one side of the head there may be postnatal development of plagiocephaly. Again, this may be distinguished from postnatal constraint deformation by the history.

References

1. Dunn, P. M.: Congenital sternomastoid torticollis: An intrauterine postural deformity. Arch. Dis. Child. *49*:824, 1974.
2. Clarren, S. K., Smith, D. W., and Hanson, J. W.: Helmet treatment for plagiocephaly and congenital muscular torticollis. J. Pediatr. *94*:43, 1979.
3. Clarren, S. K.: Plagiocephaly and torticollis: Etiology, natural history, and helmet treatment. J. Pediatr. *98*:92, 1981.
4. Jones, M. C.: Unilateral epicanthal fold: Diagnostic significance. J. Pediatr. *108*:702, 1986.
5. Aase, J. M.: Structural defects as a consequence of late intrauterine constraint: Craniotabies, loose skin, and asymmetric ear size. Sem. Perinatol. 7:270, 1983.
6. Jones, P. G.: Torticollis in Infancy and Childhood. Sternomastoid Fibrosis and the Sternomastoid "Tumour." Springfield, IL, Charles C Thomas, 1968.
7. von Reuss, A. R.: The Diseases of the Newborn. New York, William Wood and Co., 1921.
8. Brooks, B.: Pathologic changes in muscle as a result of disturbances of circulation. Arch. Surg. 5:188, 1922.
9. Donahue, K. C., Charman, C. E., Chaisson, R., and Graham, J. M., Jr.: Postnatal head deformation: Anthropological observations and applications to the treatment of postnatal plagiocephaly. Am. J. Med. Genet., in press, 1987.
10. Dingwall, E. J.: Artificial Cranial Deformations: A Contribution to the Study of Ethnic Mutilation. London, John Bale, Sons, & Danielsson, Ltd., 1931.

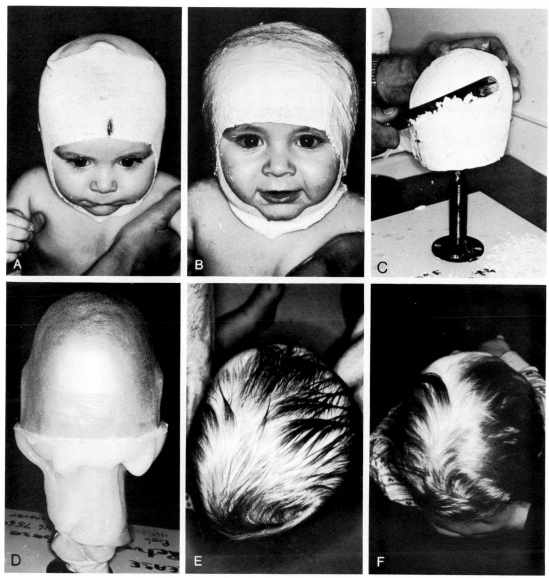

Figure 2–23. *A* and *B,* Following the procedures outlined by Clarren[2, 3] when conservative measures proved unsuccessful in correcting this child's plagiocephaly by age six months, a stockinette cap was placed over the infant's head to prevent hair from becoming embedded in the rapidly drying plaster splint material. *C,* Plaster of Paris is poured into the mold, and an iron pipe is placed in the bust, which is then allowed to dry overnight. The mold is removed, and the bust is mounted on a base so that it can be molded into a symmetrical shape. Where the bust is flattened and continuing brain growth is wanted to fill out the calvarium, plaster is added to the bust. In areas that are too prominent, the bust is left unchanged. Foam to pad the inside of the helmet is stretched around the augmented bust, to which ear spaces have been added. The foam is stretched around the bust in two layers separated by talcum powder, and then 3/8-inch polypropylene plastic is molded around the bust in a vacuum oven. *D,* The helmet is cut off the bust, and the infant wears the helmet constantly (except for baths) until it will not fit any longer. *E,* Before helmet therapy was begun at six months, there was asymmetrical occipital flattening, which resolved by nine months *(F).*

Illustration continued on following page

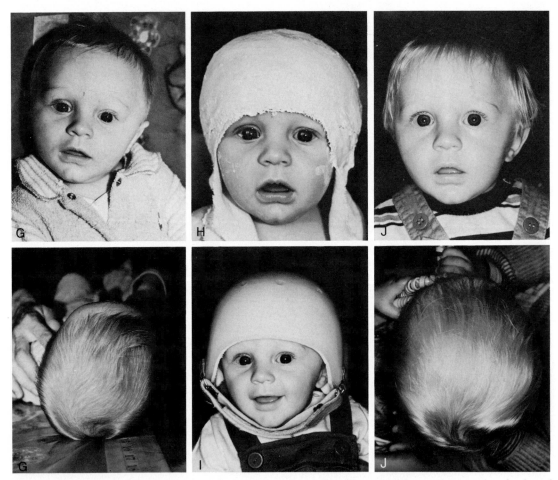

Figure 2–23 *Continued. G,* This infant was born to a small primigravida woman by cesarean section for breech presentation. He had the plagiocephaly-torticollis deformation sequence with residual calvarial asymmetry at six months. *H,* Rapidly drying splint material was used to make a mold of his aberrant head shape. *I,* He wore the helmet for the next six months, with partial correction occurring by age 10 months *(J).*

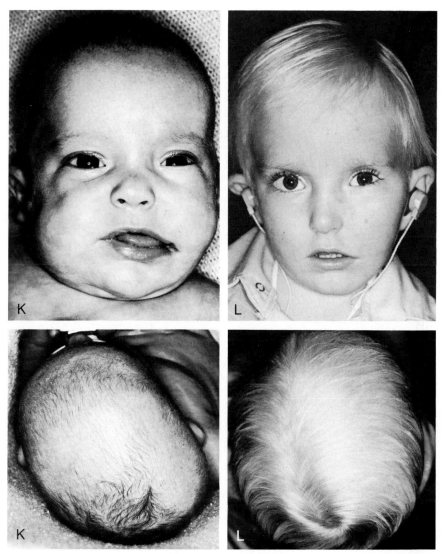

Figure 2–23 *Continued. K* and *L*, This infant with oculoauricular vertebral dysplasia had severe cervical vertebral anomalies that resulted in a persistent head turn to the right. By age three months *(K)*, he had developed marked plagiocephaly as a consequence of his asymmetrical resting position. Because the cervical vertebral anomalies could not be corrected, he was fitted with two consecutive helmets to maintain normal cranial symmetry during the period of most rapid head growth (through two years of age). At three years of age *(L)*, he had persistent head turn and head tilt but relatively normal cranial symmetry.

Illustration continued on following page

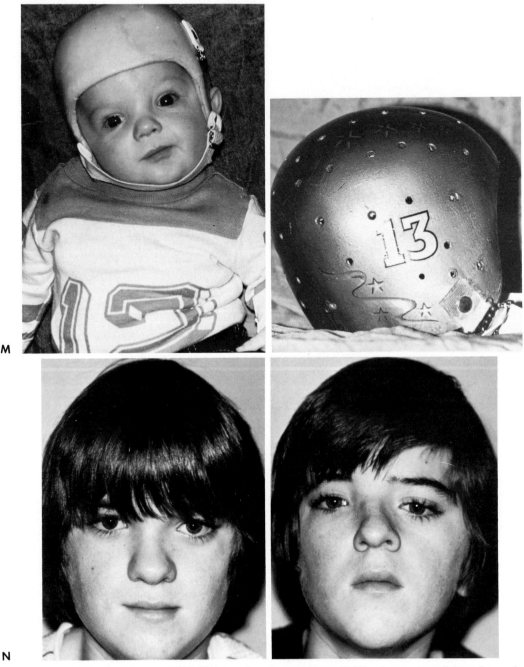

Figure 2–23 *Continued. M*, We supply the helmets, but the rest is supplied by the parents of these future football players of America! *N*, Although most mild degrees of plagiocephaly with torticollis will resolve spontaneously, permanent deformation can result, as shown in these 10-year-old monozygotic twins who are not "identical" because one incurred a greater degree of in-utero head molding than the other. (*G* through *J* adapted from Graham, J. M., Jr.: Alterations in head shape as a consequence of fetal head constraint. Sem. Perinatol. 7:257, 1983.)

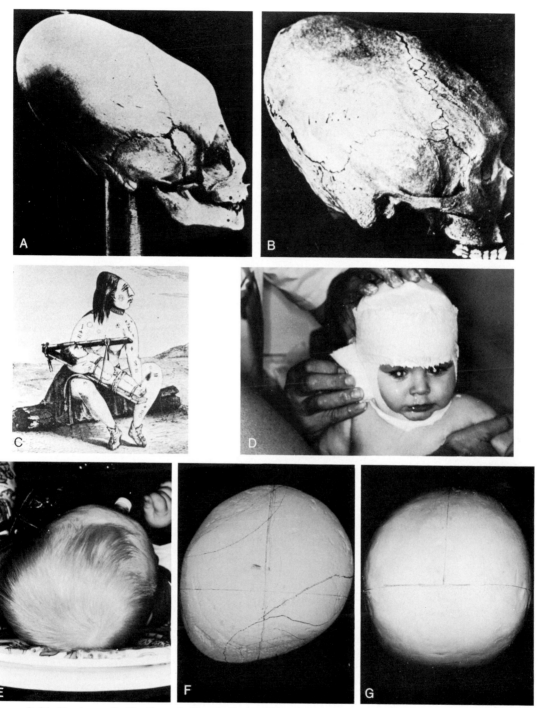

Figure 2–24. Northwest Pacific Coast Indian skulls (*A*, Chinook; *B*, Kwakiutl) demonstrate the consequences of purposeful cranial deformation during infancy. *C*, They applied boards to the occiput and frontal regions from birth until the child walked. Taking a cue from these practices, we can make helmets that allow an infant's head to grow into a symmetrical shape. *D*, This process begins by making a mold of the infant's asymmetrical head and then augmenting the bust to create a symmetrical shape from which a helmet is made. *E*, An infant with torticollis who spent prolonged periods in a rigid infant seat inadvertently molded his head into an asymmetrical shape. *F*, Viewed from the top, these figures demonstrate the uncorrected *(F)* and corrected *(G)* busts for the infant in *E*, who responded nicely to helmet therapy. (*A* through *C* adapted from Dingwall, E. J.: Artificial Cranial Deformation. A Contribution to the Study of Ethnic Mutilation. London, John Bale, Sons, and Danielsson, Ltd., 1931.)

11.0 CRANIOSTENOSIS, GENERAL

GENESIS. Limitation of the normal growth stretch at a suture during fetal life may result in craniostenosis. This has been shown to occur, for example, when the lack of growth stretch is caused by a deficit in brain growth, as in severe primary microcephaly. Experimental prolongation of gestation, resulting in fetal crowding after installation of a cervical clip in pregnant mice, has been shown to result in craniosynostosis.[1] The most common cause of craniostenosis in the human is considered to be constraint of the fetal head in utero (Fig. 2–25).[2–6] The external constraint limits growth stretch in the direction between the constraining points and may cause craniostenosis of an intervening suture. The constrained suture tends to develop a bony ridge, especially at the point of maximal constraint. This will prevent future growth at that site, and the expanding brain will then distort the calvarium into aberrant shape.

FEATURES. The features are dependent on which sutures are stenotic, the extent of craniostenosis, and the timing of the problem. The earlier the craniostenosis occurs, the more profound is its impact on subsequent craniofacial and brain development. Craniostenosis of multiple sutures may limit overall brain growth and result in increased intracranial pressure.[7] On roentgenograms, the cranial vault, which is under increased pressure because of craniostenosis, tends to have a "beaten silver" appearance. The precise reason for this phenomenon is not known, but it may be the result of altered magnitude and direction of forces on the bony trabecular organization within the calvarium.

MANAGEMENT AND PROGNOSIS. Mild degrees of craniostenosis may not merit treatment. However, in moderate to severe cases, early surgical therapy is usually warranted. Except for instances in which both coronal and sagittal sutures are stenotic, impairing brain growth, the predominant indication for surgery is cosmetic restoration of normal shape. A variety of neurosurgical techniques have been developed for the treatment of craniostenosis.[8] Most of these techniques involve removing the aberrant portion of the bony calvarium from its underlying dura, including the area surrounding the stenotic suture(s). If this is done within the first few months after birth a new bony calvarium will usually develop within the remaining dura mater under the same principles that normally guide calvarial morphogenesis;[10] namely, that intradural mineralization begins between the sites of dural reflection. As long as there is continued growth stretch from the expanding brain, the sites over the dural reflections remain unossified, thereby forming the sutures. Thus the calvarium and its sutures may develop normally after a partial calvariectomy for constraint-induced craniostenosis. The new bony calvarium begins to develop within two to three weeks and is usually firm by five to eight weeks. If the procedure is done after three to four months of age, the approach is similar with the exception that pieces of the calvarium are replaced in a mosaic over the dura mater to act as niduses for mineralization of the new calvarium.

DIFFERENTIAL DIAGNOSIS. There are a number of other causes of craniostenosis.[11] These can be divided into several general categories such as problems of the brain or mesenchymal tissues and metabolic disorders.[9, 11]

Brain Problems. Basic problems in early brain morphogenesis may cause a lack of dural reflection and hence lack of a suture, thereby resulting in inability of the calvarium to grow laterally in that region.[10] Observed examples include: (1) holoprosencephaly (single ventricle) with no anterior interhemispheric fissure and consequently no metopic suture; (2) unilateral deficiency of the early cerebrum with no insular sulcus and hence no sphenoid wing or its dural reflection and thus no coronal suture. Deficit of brain growth, such as in severe microcephaly, may result in a lack of expansile brain force with craniostenosis as a secondary consequence. More localized brain growth deficiency may cause a particular suture to become prematurely craniostenotic. For example, frontal brain growth deficiency may result in metopic craniostenosis. Excessive shunting of hydrocephalus may also cause a lack of growth stretch at the suture lines, enhancing the tendency toward craniostenosis.[9]

Mesenchymal Tissue Problems. There are a number of disorders in which craniostenosis appears to occur because of an aberration in mesenchymal tissues. One such example, Apert syndrome, features not only craniostenosis but also osseous syndactyly. Most of these disorders are genetically determined.

Metabolic Problems. Early rickets, regardless of its cause, is strangely liable to result in craniosynostosis. In rare instances early hyperthyroidism also has been a cause, as has hypercalcemia.[9]

References

1. Koskinen-Moffett, L.: In vivo experimental model for prenatal craniostenosis. J. Dent. Res. *65*:special issue, Abstr. 980, 1986.
2. Graham, J. M., Jr., deSaxe, M., and Smith, D. W.: Sagittal craniostenosis: Fetal head constraint as one possible cause. J. Pediatr. *95*:747, 1979.
3. Graham, J. M., Jr., Badura, R., and Smith, D. W.: Coronal craniostenosis: Fetal head constraint as one possible cause. Pediatrics *65*:995, 1980.
4. Graham, J. M., Jr., and Smith, D. W.: Metopic craniostenosis and fetal head constraint: Two interesting experiments of nature. Pediatrics *65*:1000, 1980.
5. Higginbottom, M. C., Jones, K. L., and James, H. E.: Intrauterine constraint and craniosynostosis. Neurosurgery *6*:39, 1980.
6. Graham, J. M., Jr.: Alterations in head shape as a consequence of fetal head constraint. Sem. Perinatol. *7*:257, 1983.
7. Renier, D., Sainte-Rose, C., Marchac, D., and Hirsch, J.-F.: Intracranial pressure in craniostenosis. J. Neurosurg. *57*:370, 1982.
8. Hanson, J. W., Sayers, J. P., Knopp, L. M., Mac-Donald, C., and Smith, D. W.: Total neonatal calvariectomy for severe craniosynstosis. J. Pediatr. *91*:257, 1977.
9. Cohen, M. M., Jr. (Ed.): Craniosynostosis: Diagnosis, Evaluation, and Management. New York, Raven Press, 1986.
10. Smith, D. W., and Töndury, G.: Origins of the calvarium and its sutures. Am. J. Dis. Child. *132*:662, 1978.
11. Freeman, J. M., and Borkowf, S.: Craniostenosis: Review of the literature and report of thirty-four cases. Pediatrics *30*:57, 1962.

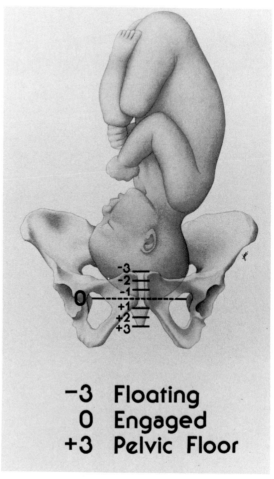

Figure 2–25. Craniostenosis, general. The head may become engaged in the pelvis in such a manner as to limit lateral growth at the sagittal suture. This is considered to be a factor that can enhance the risk of sagittal craniostenosis. (Courtesy of Jan A. Norbisrath, Medical Illustrator, Obstetrics and Gynecology, University of Washington Medical School.)

11.1 Craniostenosis, Sagittal

GENESIS. Early descent of the fetal head into the maternal pelvis, often four weeks or more before delivery, with fetal head entrapment resulting in biparietal constraint is considered the most common cause of sagittal craniostenosis.[1, 2] This mode of genesis is shown in Figure 2–26. The sagittal ridging tends to be most prominent at the site between the parietal eminences, where theoretically lateral constraint would be maximized. The platypelloid pelvis, relatively small in the anterior-posterior compared with the lateral dimensions, would hypothetically constitute the greatest risk for this type of entrapment head constraint. Sagittal craniostenosis is the most common type of craniostenosis, occurring about once in 2000 births. It has a 3:1 predilection for males. This has been attributed to the more rapid rate of head growth in the male during the last trimester of gestation.[1, 2] The larger head is simply more likely to become seriously constrained.

FEATURES. The head is long and narrow (dolichocephalic) with a prominent forehead and occiput. There is a ridge along the mid to posterior sagittal suture that is most prominent between the biparietal eminences (scaphocephaly). The relatively excessive anterior-posterior growth may partially spread the coronal and/or lambdoidal sutures, and restraint of growth along the posterior sagittal suture may result in flattening between the occiput and the vertex. The head circumference may be spuriously increased, providing a mistaken impression of macrocephaly or even hydrocephaly. Examination of the synostotic suture histologically reveals complete obliteration of the sutural ligament with endocranial bone resorption and ectocranial bone deposition.[3]

MANAGEMENT, PROGNOSIS AND COUNSEL. (See also the section on general craniostenosis.) Craniostenosis of the sagittal suture alone imposes a moderate cosmetic problem. It may sometimes be difficult for the parents and physician to resolve the question as to whether or not surgical intervention is indicated. One woman who never had surgery experienced severe pressure-type headaches at 13 to 15 years of age. In retrospect, these were interpreted as having been secondary to increased intracranial pressure during her adolescent brain growth spurt at a time when the other sutures were unable to completely accommodate to the problem of the sagittal craniostenosis.

Partial calvariectomy should include all of the sagittal suture region and a wide zone to either side. For the best cosmetic results, the bony calvarium of the occipital and bregmal promontories may be excised; these promontories will not recur.

Most constraint-induced instances of sagittal craniostenosis are sporadic; however, it has not been determined whether some rare instances of familial sagittal craniostenosis are a consequence of inherited pelvic type, or are part of a broader pattern of heritable malformation.

References

1. Graham, J. M., Jr., deSaxe, M., and Smith, D. W.: Sagittal craniostenosis: Fetal head constraint as one possible cause. J. Pediatr. 95:747, 1979.
2. Graham, J. M., Jr.: Alterations in head shape as a consequence of fetal head constraint. Sem. Perinatol. 7:257, 1983.
3. Koskinen-Moffett, L. K., Moffett, B. C., Jr., and Graham, J. M., Jr.: Cranial synostosis and intrauterine compression: A developmental study of human sutures. In Dixon, A. D., and Sarnat, B. G. (eds.): Factors and Mechanisms Influencing Bone Growth. New York, Alan R. Liss, 1982, pp. 365–378.

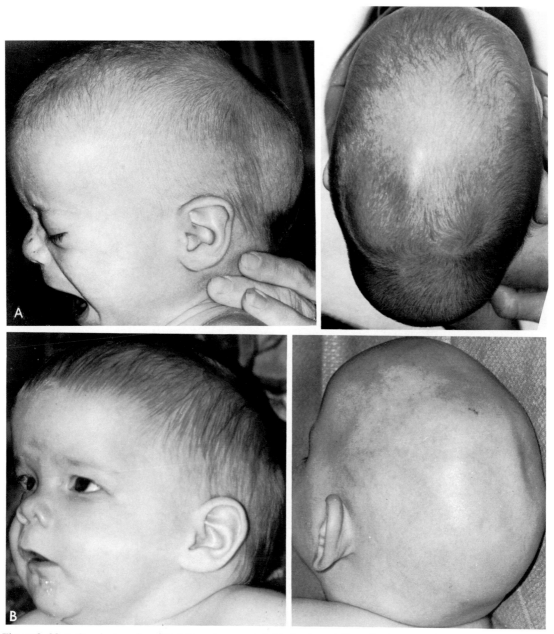

Figure 2–26. *A*, Craniostenosis, sagittal. Prominent occipital bulge in an infant who has posterior sagittal craniostenosis, with palpable ridging at the site of craniosynostosis. *B*, Early descent of the fetal head into the pelvis may limit the lateral growth stretch at the sagittal suture line, resulting in craniostenosis. Note the prominent forehead with the scaphocephalic head. Ridging of the sagittal suture was most prominently evident at the area between the biparietal sites of presumed in-utero constraint of lateral head growth.

Illustration continued on following page

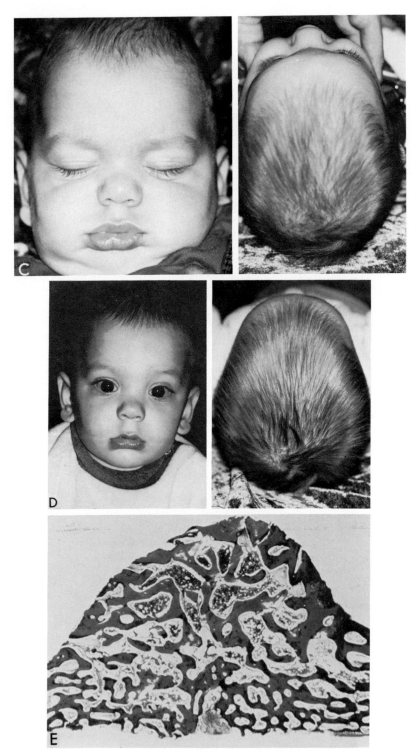

Figure 2–26 *Continued. C,* Infant with sagittal craniostenosis. Note the relatively narrow biparietal diameter of the scaphocephalic head. *D,* Same infant at nine months of age, following partial calvariectomy with correction of sagittal craniostenosis. Note the dramatic change in the bifrontal versus biparietal dimensions in the top view of the head. *E,* Histology shows ridged synostotic suture with resorption of bone at inner table of the calvarium at the site between the usual parietal eminences.

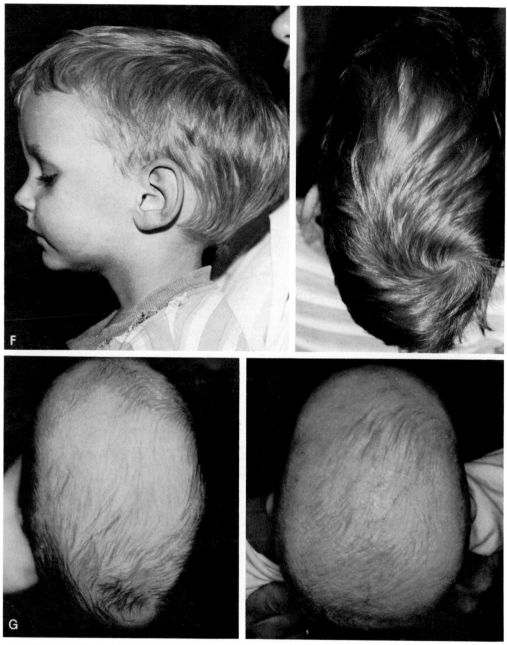

Figure 2–26 *Continued. F,* Six-year-old with unoperated sagittal craniostenosis (note scaphocephaly with prominent occipital bulge). *G,* One-month-old infant with unoperated sagittal craniostenosis (left) showing similar head shape to *F.* This head shape resolved (right) by 3½ months (10 weeks after surgery).

11.2 Craniostenosis, Coronal

GENESIS. Constraint-induced coronal craniostenosis can be secondary to early descent of the fetal head into a constraining pelvis, to an aberrant fetal lie, or to constraint within a bicornuate uterus.[1-3] The left side is more commonly affected than the right, and this has been ascribed to the LOA birth position, which tends to result in more coronal constraint on the left side than on the right.[1] The coronal stenosis secondarily affects the anterior craniofacies, as shown in Figure 2–27.

FEATURES. With bilateral coronal craniostenosis, the forehead is high (oxycephaly) and broad, resulting in a head that is short (brachycephaly). The impact of the coronal stenosis on the craniofacies is summarized in Figure 2–27. When it is unilateral, the impact on the facies is unilateral, and the face may appear asymmetric. Within the skull the sphenoid ridge tends to be high and thickened.

MANAGEMENT, PROGNOSIS, AND COUNSEL. The cosmetic impact of coronal craniostenosis is of such magnitude that early surgical intervention is generally warranted. Furthermore, the child with untreated coronal stenosis has a small nasopharynx that tends to foster middle ear infection and an abnormal oral cavity that contributes to both speech problems and dental malocclusion. The partial calvariectomy for coronal stenosis should start behind the area of the coronal suture and extend well below the suture laterally. The bony resection should be extended to include the bony sphenoid ridges as far medially as feasible and frontally to include the brow and the orbital roofs (prior to four months of age). Often, bony struts are wired in place to help advance the orbits. The brain may then move forward and model the new anterior calvarium. Furthermore, the cranial base, which is the roof of the face, can grow forward, carrying the midface with it. Thus, the secondary craniofacial aspects of coronal craniostenosis can be largely re-formed toward a more normal appearance. However, to accomplish this, the surgery should ideally be done in early infancy. The forward growth of the cranial base is 56 per cent complete by birth and 70 per cent complete by two years of age. With malformation syndromes that limit the growth of the anterior cranial base, surgery will be less effective in restoring normal facial features.

DIFFERENTIAL DIAGNOSIS. The sequence of coronal synostosis may occur by itself or as part of an autosomal dominant disorder usually referred to as Crouzon syndrome. It may also occur in a number of other syndromes, such as Apert syndrome, Pfeiffer syndrome, or Saethre-Chotzen syndrome, in which various types of limb anomalies are also present.

Constraint limitation of craniofacial growth may occasionally yield an appearance at birth that is quite similar to that of coronal stenosis and its consequences, *except* that craniosynostosis is not found at the time of early surgery. Such patients demonstrate rapid spontaneous restitution toward normal form in the first few postnatal weeks, which would not be expected with coronal stenosis. For this one reason it is probably best to wait several weeks or longer before making a decision about calvarial surgery unless the problem is severe with evidence of increased intracranial pressure.

References

1. Graham, J. M., Jr., Badura, R., and Smith, D. W.: Coronal craniostenosis: Fetal head constraint as one possible cause. Pediatrics 65:995, 1980.
2. Higginbottom, M. C., Jones, K. L., and James, H. E.: Intrauterine constraint and craniosynostosis. Neurosurgery 6:39, 1980.
3. Graham, J. M., Jr.: Alterations in head shape as a consequence of fetal head constraint. Sem. Perinatol. 7:257, 1983.

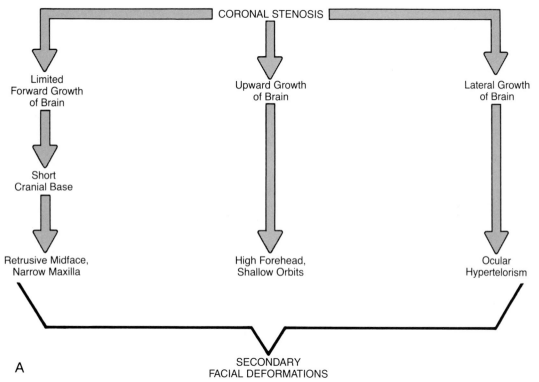

Figure 2–27. Craniostenosis, coronal. *A,* Coronal craniostenosis in early life appears to result in secondary facial deformations.

Illustration continued on following page

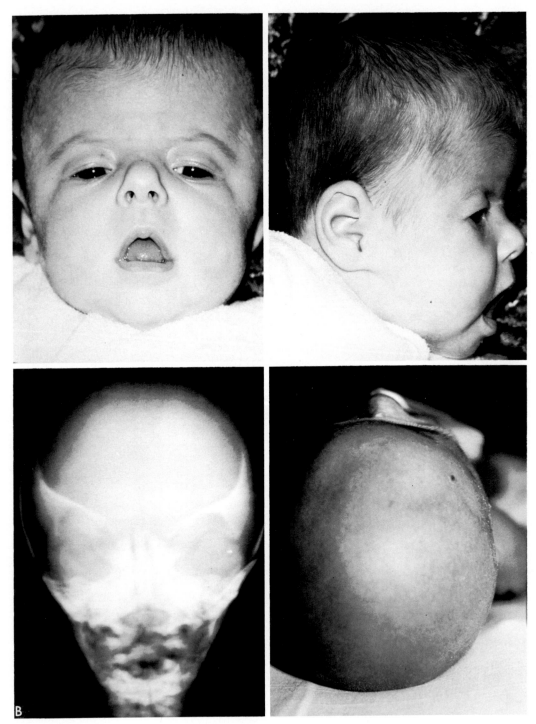

Figure 2–27 *Continued. B,* Bilateral coronal craniostenosis in a young infant with secondary facial deformations, short brachycephalic head, and "harlequin" radiographic sign caused by upward flare of the sphenoidal ridges.

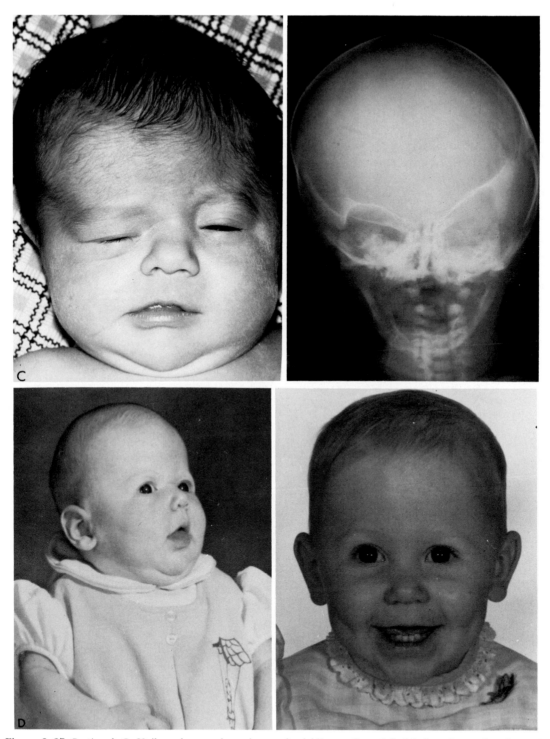

Figure 2–27 *Continued. C,* Unilateral coronal craniostenosis yielding unilateral facial distortion and radiographic harlequin sign. *D,* Early surgical intervention at several months (left) of the coronal craniostenosis (by Dr. Nelson) allowed the mid-face to move forward to yield a normal facies by 14 months (right).

Illustration continued on following page

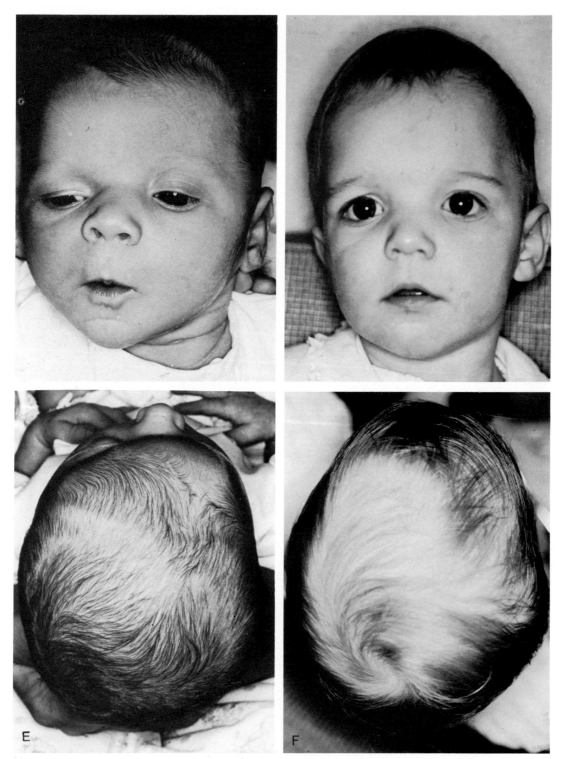

Figure 2–27 *Continued. E,* At nine days this infant demonstrated palpable ridging over her synostotic left coronal suture. *F,* Frontal calvariectomy at six weeks of age (by Dr. Dick Saunders) resulted in a complete restoration of normal features that persisted, as demonstrated here by similar head views at age 17 months.

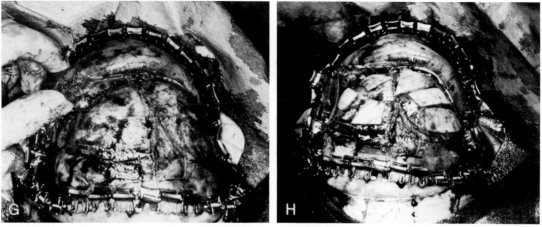

Figure 2–27 *Continued. G* and *H,* Operative photographs of the patient in *E* and *F,* viewed from the top of the head with the nose toward the top of the figure. Exposure of the calvarium *(G)* reveals a synostotic left coronal suture with restriction of the left frontal region. The left orbit is advanced with a bony strut *(H),* and pieces of calvarium are used as a mosaic to facilitate reformation of new cranial bone. *(E* through *H* adapted from Graham, J. M., Jr.: Alterations in head shape as a consequence of fetal head constraint. Sem. Perinatol. 7:257, 1983.)

11.3 Craniostenosis, Lambdoidal

GENESIS. Lambdoidal craniostenosis accounts for less than 5 per cent of all cases of craniostenosis. It can result from constraint of the posterior cranium associated with abnormal fetal lie or presentation.

FEATURES. Unilateral synostosis results in plagiocephaly, whereas bilateral involvement leads to brachycephaly. Unlike coronal synostosis, facial structures and orbits are usually not seriously affected, although unilateral involvement results in ipsilateral occipital flattening and anterior displacement of the pinna (Fig. 2–28). Radiographic signs include cranial asymmetry, small posterior fossa, and sutural sclerosis.

MANAGEMENT AND PROGNOSIS. Because isolated lambdoidal synostosis is usually not associated with elevations in intracranial pressure, posterior calvariectomy is done for cosmetic reasons in severely affected cases. The timing for such surgery can be later than for other forms of craniostenosis, and the response to surgery is usually less dramatic.

DIFFERENTIAL DIAGNOSIS. As with other forms of craniostenosis, the primary consideration should be to determine whether lambdoidal craniostenosis is isolated or part of a broader pattern of altered morphogenesis. It can occur in children with chromosome anomalies.[2] For children with isolated unilateral lambdoidal craniostenosis, it may be difficult to determine whether the suture is synostotic or simply overlapping. Infants with ipsilateral occipital flattening, anterior displacement of the pinna, and torticollis may be treated with helmet therapy if there is no sutural synostosis (see 10. Oblique Head Deformation: Plagiocephaly-Torticollis Sequence).

References

1. Cohen, M. M., Jr. (Ed.): Craniosynostosis: Diagnosis, Evaluation, and Management. New York, Raven Press, 1986.
2. Park, J. P., Wurster-Hill, D. H., Berg, S. Z., and Graham, J. M., Jr.: A denovo interstitial deletion of chromosome 6 (q22.2 p23.1), Clin. Genet. in press, 1987.

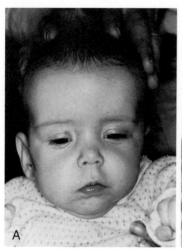 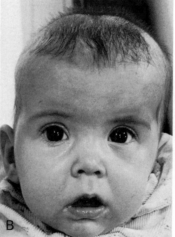 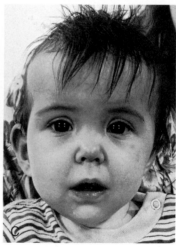

Figure 2–28. This child was delivered by cesarean section from a persistent transverse lie. *A*, She had mild facial asymmetry prior to surgery at three months. *B*, One month after the operation the facial asymmetry had improved, and further improvement was evident five months postoperatively *(C)*.

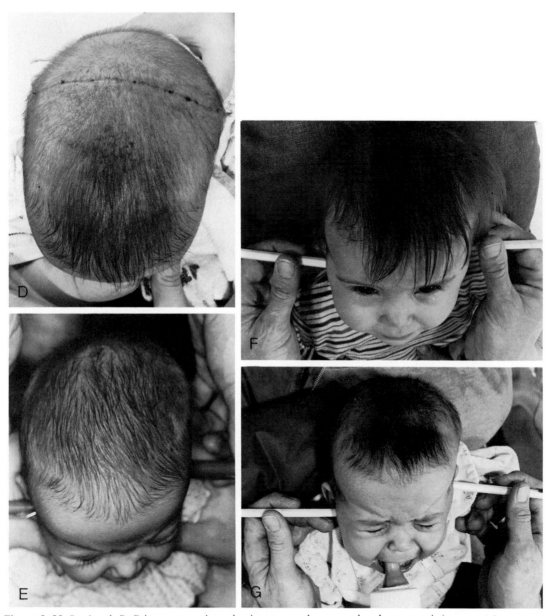

Figure 2–28 *Continued. D,* Prior to posterior calvariectomy at three months, there was obvious cranial asymmetry (plagiocephaly) with ridging and hyperostosis of the right lambdoid suture. *E,* One month postoperatively, cranial asymmetry was improved. *F,* Particularly evident prior to surgery was the relative advancement of the right ear versus the left. *G,* Positioning of the ears had improved by five months after the operation, as shown by the pencils positioned at the external auditory canals.

11.4 Craniostenosis, Metopic

GENESIS. Lateral constraint of the frontal part of the head may cause early metopic craniostenosis (Fig. 2–29). Examples have included one of MZ triplets whose forehead had been wedged between the buttocks of her two sisters in utero and an infant whose head had been "impacted" in a bicornuate uterine horn.[1]

FEATURES. There is a narrow and sometimes prow-shaped forehead with a ridged metopic suture. There may be secondary upslanting to the palpebral fissures and ocular hypotelorism.

MANAGEMENT AND PROGNOSIS. Generally, no treatment is utilized in mild cases with no associated deformity. Moderate to severe instances often warrant a frontal calvariectomy, ideally including the entire forehead down to the supraorbital ridges. In the more severe cases that include hypotelorism, the brows and orbital roofs should also be removed.

DIFFERENTIAL DIAGNOSIS. It is important to exclude primary defects of brain, such as the holoprosencephaly malformation complex and the Opitz trigonocephaly syndrome.[2] The latter condition includes unusual facial features, hypotonia, multiple frenula, limb defects, visceral anomalies, mental deficiency, and probable autosomal recessive inheritance. Metopic craniostenosis can also accompany a variety of chromosomal abnormalities, particularly deletions of the long arm of chromosome 11.[2]

References

1. Graham, J. M., Jr., and Smith, D. W.: Metopic craniostenosis as a consequence of fetal head constraint: Two interesting experiments of nature. Pediatrics 65:1000, 1980.
2. Cohen, M. M., Jr. (Ed.): Craniosynostosis: Diagnosis, Evaluation and Management. New York, Raven Press, 1986.

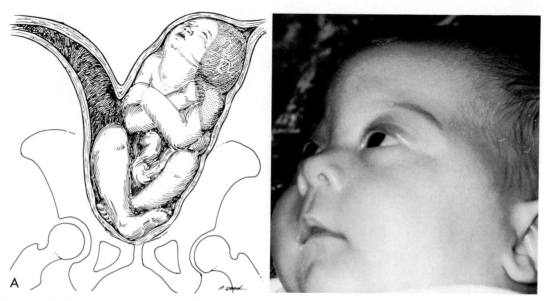

Figure 2–29. Craniostenosis, metopic. *A*, Metopic craniostenosis in an infant who was reared in a bicornuate uterus. At cesarean section it required several minutes to dislodge the head from its tightly entrapped position in one upper uterine horn.

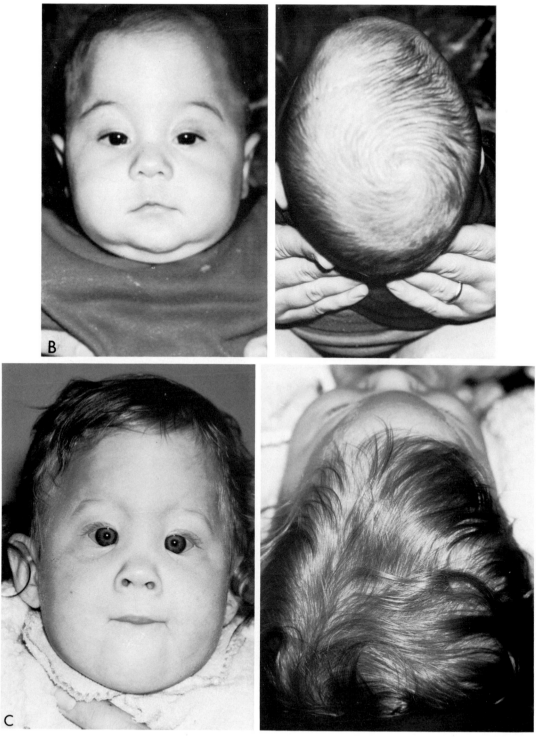

Figure 2–29 *Continued. B,* Postoperative status of the infant shown in *A* following calvariectomy of the frontal bone region down to the supraorbital ridges, allowing the brain to remold the forehead as a more normally shaped bony calvarium was formed. *C,* One of monozygotic triplets reared in a 104-pound woman who gained 64 pounds during the pregnancy. Roentgenograms had shown the patient to have the frontal portion of her head wedged between the buttocks of her co-triplets. This was considered the source of the constraint that yielded the metopic craniostenosis with secondary narrow forehead and upslanting palpebral fissures, features that were not shared by her monozygotic co-triplets. (From Graham, J. M., Jr., and Smith, D. W.: Metopic craniostenosis as a consequence of fetal head constraint. Two interesting experiments of nature. Pediatrics *65*:1000, 1980. Reproduced by permission of Pediatrics.)

11.5 Craniostenosis: Sagittal Plus Coronal

GENESIS. Constraint as the cause of sagittal plus coronal craniostenosis is unusual and would usually be of profound degree. Restoration of normal form after surgery is more likely when constraint is the cause of the problem.

FEATURES. In this condition the limitations of calvarial expansion are so extreme that there is limited room for brain growth (Fig. 2–30). Synostosis of multiple cranial sutures is more likely to result in elevated intracranial pressure than single suture synostosis.[1] Besides the oxycephalic head shape resulting from coronal stenosis, there are usually signs of increased intracranial pressure and a "beaten silver" roentgenographic appearance of the inner table of the skull. There may also be optic atrophy, proptosis, and loss of vision. Combinations of sutural synostosis, such as sagittal plus coronal, are also referred to as compound craniosynostosis.

MANAGEMENT AND PROGNOSIS. Early extensive calvariectomy is merited to preserve brain function and development as well as to allow reformation of the craniofacial skeletal features.[2]

DIFFERENTIAL DIAGNOSIS. This degree of craniostenosis is more commonly found in some of the genetically determined disorders, such as Crouzon syndrome, Apert syndrome, Pfeiffer syndrome, or Saethre-Chotzen syndrome.

References

1. Renier, D., Sainte-Rose, C., Marchac, D., and Hirsh, J.-F.: Intrauterine pressure in craniostenosis. J. Neurosurg. 57:370, 1982.
2. Hanson, J. W., Sayer, M. P., Knopp, L. M., Macdonald, C., and Smith, D. W.: Subtotal neonatal calvariectomy for severe craniosynostosis. J. Pediatr. 91:257, 1977.

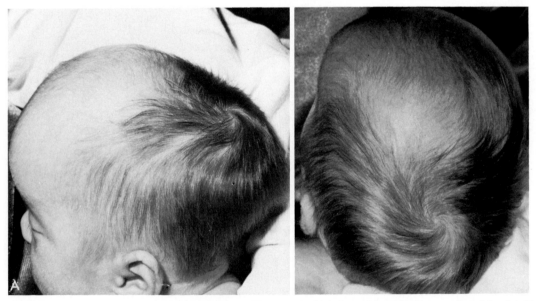

Figure 2–30. Craniostenosis, sagittal plus coronal. *A,* Three-week-old infant with sagittal, coronal, and lambdoidal craniosynostosis. Only the metopic suture was open and the brain growth ballooned out into this region, which was under increased pressure. The coronal synostosis plus the bulging forehead region had distorted the mid and upper facies. A calvariectomy was performed by Dr. Peter Sayers from the supraorbital ridge to below the coronal suture, above the mastoid and above the foramen magnum. The aberrant calvarium was discarded, and within several weeks a new calvarium was forming from the remaining dura mater.

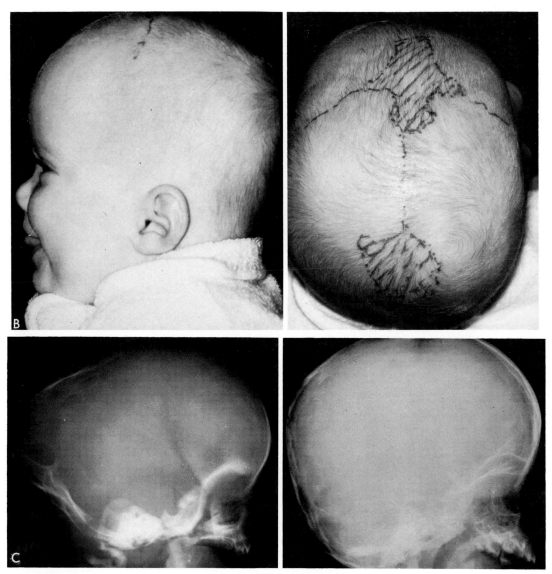

Figure 2–30 *Continued. B,* The infant in *A* two months after calvariectomy. The brain of normal size and shape has been the guiding force in the shape of the upper head as the new calvarium has formed. The new calvarium has functional sutures at the sites of dural reflection and fontanels where the sutures join. *C,* Radiograph of the above infant before calvariectomy and after the new calvarium has formed. (*A, B,* and *C* are from Hanson, J. W., Sayer, M.P., Knopp, L. M., Macdonald, C., and Smith, D. W.: Subtotal neonatal calvariectomy for severe craniosynostosis. J. Pediatr. *91*:257–269, 1977.)

12. VERTEX BIRTH MOLDING

GENESIS. In the normal fetus presenting in the vertex position there may be appreciable molding of the head at birth, especially if he or she is the first born, is a large baby, or if the mother has a prolonged labor, has a small pelvic outlet, and/or has an incompletely dilated rigid cervix.

The following is a tentative reconstruction of how molding normally occurs. During the initial cervical dilation there is some decrease in the biparietal diameter, with a prominence and increased height of the vertex. With incomplete cervical dilation the biparietal diameter is decreased further, and there is increasing angulation toward the presenting part. The occipital bone rotates inward on the "occipital hinge," and the frontal bones bend inward. The result is a decrease in the anterior-posterior diameter (Fig. 2–31A).

FEATURES. The forehead tends to slope and the parieto-occipital region is prominent. Overlapping of sagittal, coronal, and/or lambdoidal sutures is frequent. Head circumference measurements may be spuriously low because of the nature of the molding. The head circumference may shift upward by one to three days after birth as the head remolds in relation to the true brain shape. The head usually shifts back to the original unmolded form by six days after birth (Fig. 2–31B).

Occasionally there may be a traumatic subperiosteal hemorrhage, most commonly in the outer table of the parietal bone. This will give rise to a soft, fluctuant circular mass. With time, its borders will become elevated and crater-like, as the raised periosteum begins to deposit bone at its borders. At the leading part of the parieto-occipital region there may be edema of the skin and subcutaneous tissues, the so-called caput succedaneum. Craniotabes may also be extensive in the vertex region (Fig. 2–31D). Hemorrhages may occasionally be evident in the sclerae and in the retina.

PROGNOSIS. The prognosis for spontaneous resolution of vertex birth molding and the traumatic components that may accompany it is generally excellent, and no therapy is necessary other than reassurance that the baby is normal.

DIFFERENTIAL DIAGNOSIS. A spuriously small occipitofrontal head circumference may give a mistaken impression of varying degrees of microcephaly, as may the sloping forehead. Clinical judgment about the apparent overall brain size plus follow-up head circumference measurement as the calvarium returns toward a normal shape will usually resolve any questions in this regard.

The subperiosteal hemorrhage with a subsequent crater-rim of bone at its outer borders may give the impression of a skull fracture, sometimes raising the question of a depressed skull fracture. This subperiosteal hemorrhage is a benign lesion and does *not* merit skull roentgenograms or other investigative study.

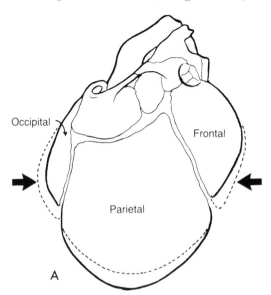

Figure 2–31. Vertex molding. *A,* Nature of forces molding the head during vertex vaginal delivery. The dashed lines show the former contour and the solid lines show the molded contour as the A-P distance is decreased while the head is increased.

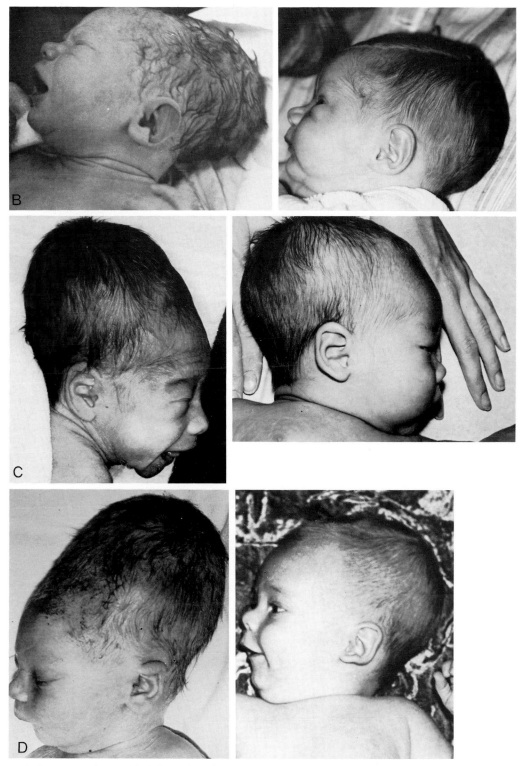

Figure 2–31 *Continued. B,* This infant showed marked molding immediately after being born (left) to a small primigravida woman. By five days of age (right), the molding had completely resolved. *C,* This infant at birth (left) had been in prolonged vertex presentation. By two months of age (right), the molding had resolved. *D,* Extreme molding (left), presumably due to a tight cervix that did not fully dilate with the delivery of this large baby. The conical vertex was palpably softened (craniotabes). The same baby is shown at 12 weeks of age (right), with complete resolution of craniotabes.

13. VERTEX CRANIOTABES

("Soft Head")

GENESIS AND FEATURES. Prolonged forceful pressure on the presenting part, usually the parieto-occipital vertex region, may result in diminished mineralization in the compressed region. This is more likely to occur in a first born, a large baby, and/or when the maternal pelvic outlet is small. The history often shows that the fetus has dropped (lightening) early and has been in the vertex position within the pelvis for an unusually long period of time. Mild degrees of this compressional craniotabes occur in 2 per cent of newborn babies, whereas extensive degrees are less common.[1]

The parieto-occipital region tends to be soft, and often there is a craniotabes "ping-pong" feel on finger compression. In one extreme instance, the entire top of the head, an area measuring 8 × 10 cm, was involved (Fig. 2–32). The presence of a normally firm bony calvarium along the sides of the calvarium and in the mastoid regions readily differentiates this from the craniotabes that is due to a generalized problem of mineralization, such as hypophosphatasia, osteogenesis imperfecta, or rickets. Within the affected region of the calvarium the sutures and fontanels may feel wider than usual.

Accentuated vertex molding and other features noted in the foregoing section are common features. The fetus with a vertex craniotabes has often been more constrained than usual in late gestation and may have mild to moderate limitation of full movement in some joints, especially those of the lower limbs.

PROGNOSIS AND COUNSEL. The prognosis is excellent, and the parents may be reassured that the calvarium will mineralize in a normal fashion within one to two months, that there is no risk in handling the "soft head," and that no special precautions are merited.

DIFFERENTIAL DIAGNOSIS. Concern may be generated about problems of mineralization, such as hypophosphatasia, osteogenesis imperfecta, or rickets. The clinical examination of the whole calvarium will readily resolve such concern. The sides of the calvarium are of normal firmness. Furthermore, there are no problems in skeletal morphogenesis except for the vertex craniotabes. This is not an indication for roentgenograms or for serum calcium phosphorus or alkaline phosphatase studies.

The "soft head" will often convey the impression of open sutures and fontanels, and the question of hydrocephalus or other reasons for increased intracranial pressure may be raised. Such concern may be fostered by increased transillumination in the vertex region when a strong light is held at the soft portion of the calvarium. The head circumference, the head shape, the character of the sutures in the firm portion of the calvarium, and the general clinical status of the infant should resolve these concerns *without* resort to skull roentgenograms or any other studies. If there is concern about a major problem, then close clinical follow-up should resolve the situation without laboratory or roentgenographic studies, since the "soft head" due to compression will normalize postnatally.

Reference

1. Graham, J. M., and Smith, D. W.: Parietal craniotabes in the neonate: Its origin and relevance. J. Pediatr. *95*:114, 1979.

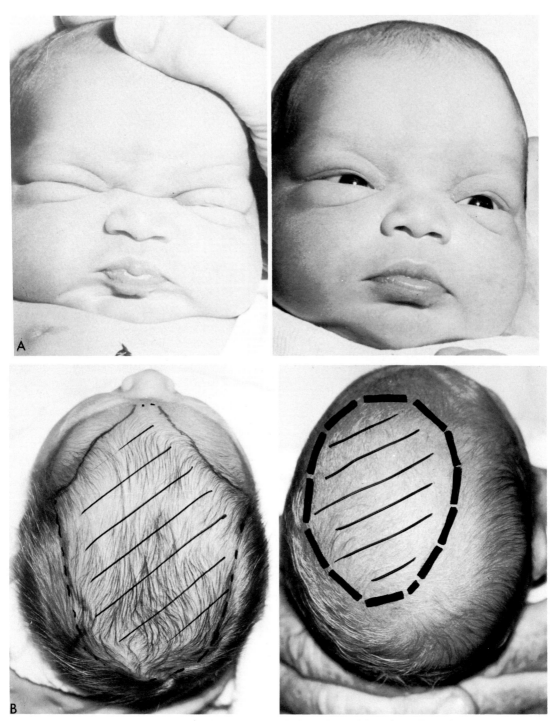

Figure 2–32. Vertex craniotabes, "soft head." *A,* Newborn infant who had been in prolonged vertex position with the head engaged under compression. Relatively forceful pressure by the examiner over the top of the head of the baby (left) did not cause discomfort, this having been the normal situation for the infant in utero. The relative excess of loose facial skin was considered an additional sign of external compression prior to birth. This baby had parietal craniotabes. The mother needs to be reassured that the appearance of the baby will improve immensely! *B,* Areas of soft "ping-pong" craniotabes, shown as hatched areas.

Illustration continued on following page

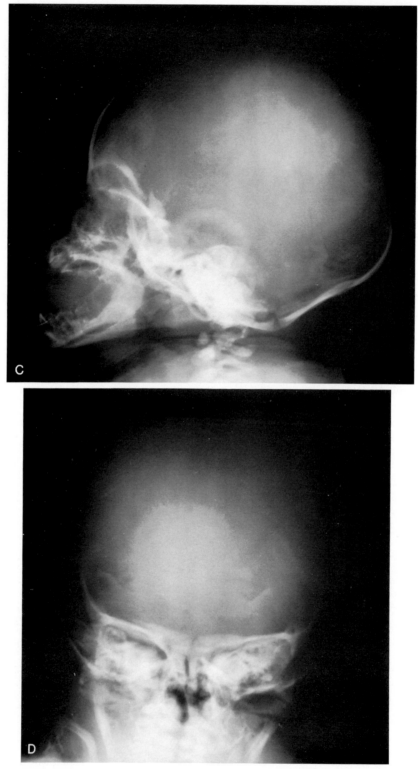

Figure 2–32 *Continued. C* and *D*, Skull radiographs from infant in *A* demonstrated diminished mineralization over the vertex. The infant's primigravida mother noted early lightening and felt the baby's head rubbing against the rim of her pelvis as she walked three miles to and from her college classes.

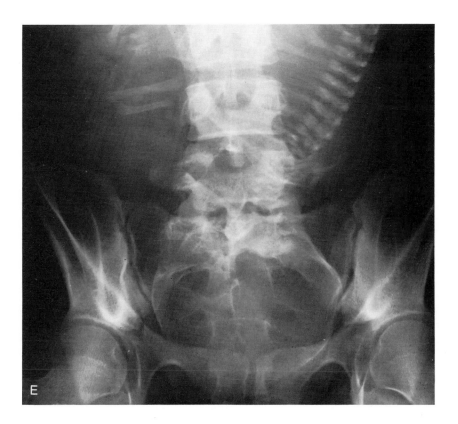

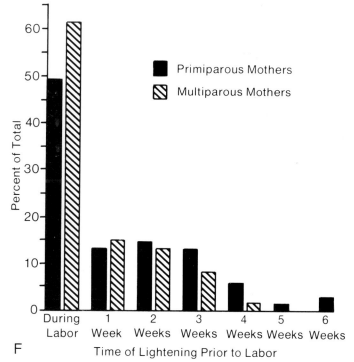

Figure 2–32 *Continued. E*, A pelvic radiograph taken two weeks prior to delivery, when her obstetrician noted fetal head engagement, demonstrates the position of the fetal head in the pelvis. *F*, Such early lightening in a primiparous mother is unusual.

14. BREECH PRESENTATION DEFORMATION

GENESIS. Breech presentation is an important cause of deformation: fully one third of deformations occur in babies who have been breech presentations.[1] Since 2 per cent of newly born babies have deformations, this indicates that 0.6 per cent of babies born have one or more deformations because of breech presentation. Therefore, this is a most important category and will be given extensive coverage.

Some of the causative factors relating to breech presentation are listed in Table 2–2. It is more common in the primigravida, especially the older woman, than in subsequent pregnancies, presumably because of the difference in the shape of the uterus and in the space for fetal and uterine growth. The spatial situation of twins in utero increases the likelihood of breech presentation, especially for the second in birth order. The prematurely born baby is still moving about in the amniotic fluid and is less likely to have shifted into the vertex birth position. Unless there is oligohydramnios, the premature fetus in breech presentation generally does not have deformations. This is because there has not been sufficient constraint to cause molding. Furthermore, as emphasized, breech presentation can be considered normal with prematurity, since at 32 weeks of gestation, 25 per cent of fetuses are in breech presentation. From this time until birth the majority of fetuses shift into vertex presentation. The frequency of breech presentation by term is 3 per cent.[1]

Any situation that causes oligohydramnios, whether it be chronic leakage of amniotic fluid or lack of urine flow into the amniotic space, will restrict movement and greatly increase the chance of the fetus being in breech presentation. Alterations of the size and shape of the uterine cavity may also increase the frequency of breech presentation. This may be secondary to a bicornuate uterus or to uterine fibroids, as two examples.

The placement of the placenta may be one factor, as emphasized by Kian[3] and summarized in Table 2–3. Placenta previa results in increased breech presentation.

About 70 per cent of fetuses in breech presentation have their legs extended in front of the abdomen.[1] Once "caught" in this position it may be most difficult for the fetus to maneuver out of this particular attitude. Tompkins[4] emphasizes that once the movements of the fetus become limited by extension of the legs in front of the abdomen, the fetus has far less chance of extricating himself or herself from the breech presentation. Dunn has made the analogy to the "folding body press" wrestling hold.[1] Once a wrestler has his opponent in this position with the legs in front of the abdomen there is little the opponent can do to extricate himself or herself.

The breech presentation with the hips flexed and knees extended is termed frank breech. With the hips and knees flexed it is called complete breech, and with hips and knees extended it is referred to as to the footling breech, as depicted in Figure 2–33A and B.

Prolonged breech position in late fetal life will give rise to uterine fundal pressure and molding of the fetal head, which may become retroflexed. This type of constraint results in anterior-posterior elongation of the head with a prominent occipital shelf, the "breech head" (Fig. 2–33C and D).[5] The shoulders are often thrust under the auricle and may also distort the mandible. The legs may be caught in front of the fetus, tending to dislocate the hips and occasionally causing genu recurvatum of the knee and often calcaneovalgus position of the feet. In the complete breech position with the legs flexed across the abdomen, the feet are liable to be compressed into an equinovarus position. The genital region, as the presenting part, may be molded and edematous.

Dunn[1] noted that 32 per cent of all deformations in the newly born baby related to breech presentation in utero. In his series of more than 6000 babies, 100 per cent of genu recurvatum cases related to breech, as did 50 per cent of hip

Table 2–2. FREQUENCY OF BREECH PRESENTATION

All pregnancies	6%
Full term singletons (highest in primigravida women)	3%
Twins	34%
Prematurely born	25%
Oligohydramnios due to chronic leakage	64%
Placenta previa	Increased
Altered shape to uterine cavity, as with bicornuate uterus	Increased
Maternal hypertension	Increased
Malformation of fetus (see Table 2–5)	Increased

Table 2–3. SITE OF IMPLANTATION AND BREECH PRESENTATION

Per Cent of All Pregnancies	Site of Implantation	Per Cent Breech
66	Cornuofundal	4
30	Midwall fundal	20
4	Midwall to low	76

dislocation cases, 42 per cent of postural scoliosis cases, and 20 to 25 per cent each for cases of mandibular asymmetry, torticollis, and talipes equinovarus. This is illustrated in Figure 2–33E.

FEATURES

Craniofacial. The head is elongated toward a scaphocephalic form, often with a prominent occipital shelf. There may be redundant folds of skin in the posterior neck, the presumed result of compression due to retroflexion of the head. The lambdoid sutures may be overlapping and/or ridged because of the fetal head constraint. The lower auricle may be forced upward into the location where the shoulder has been, and there may be a "hollow" appearance at the manubrial region of the mandible. The shoulder compression is often asymmetric, and hence there may be asymmetry of the mandible with an "upward tilt" on the more compressed side. Torticollis may occur secondary to traumatic tearing of the sternocleidomastoid muscle during vaginal delivery.

Limbs. All gradations of hip dislocation may occur in breech presentation and are considered to be the consequence of the constrained position in utero that forces the hip from its usual socket (Fig. 2–33F). The legs have generally been hyperflexed in front of the fetus, and this is often the "position of comfort" in the early neonatal period (Fig. 2–33G). As one consequence it may be difficult to fully extend and abduct the hips into the position that is usually utilized for detecting dislocation of the hips. There also may be some limitation in the full movement at the knees. This is the most common cause of genu recurvatum (Fig. 2–33H). The extended leg position may lead to calcaneovalgus foot deformity, while the flexed leg position more commonly leads to an equinovarus foot deformity (Fig. 2–33I).

Genitalia. The buttocks and genitalia tend to be the leading parts at delivery and may show edema and/or bruising (Fig. 2–33J). Secondary hydrocele of the testicle is frequent.

OTHER COMPLICATIONS OF BREECH PRESENTATION. It is important to emphasize some of the complications that can result from vaginal delivery of a baby in breech presentation. The risk of vaginal delivery must be weighed in each case against the risk of cesarean section. As more cesarean sections are being done for breech presentation, especially in the primigravida, the frequency of serious complications has fallen. Overall perinatal mortality is 13 per cent for breech presentation, much of which is accounted for by prematurely born infants, twins, and babies with malformations.[2] It is important to appreciate that the premature baby is more likely to be in the breech position in early gestation. However, it is

also important to realize that the breech position *itself* is frequently associated with premature labor. The overall frequency of breech presentation in premature deliveries from 28 to 36 weeks' gestation is 24 per cent.

For the term singleton breech without malformation the perinatal mortality is 1 per cent.[2] The breech fetus is more likely to have its head become entrapped during the second stage of labor, which tends to increase the frequency of tentorial tears and intracranial bleeding, asphyxia (five to six times greater risk), and trauma relating to the attempt to "pull" the infant out.[2] Serious consequences include trauma to the cervicothoracic nerve roots and/or brachial plexus (Klumpke's paralysis or Erb's palsy) and/or compression of the vertebral artery with cerebral ischemia.

The gravest concern is with vaginal delivery of the breech fetus who has a hyperextended head, which occurs in at least 5 per cent of breech fetuses. Of those who failed to revert to nonextended head position and were delivered by the vaginal route, 21 per cent had upper spinal cord transection.[6] The acute symptoms of such transection are usually respiratory problems, a weak cry, poor muscle tone, poor feeding, and often death. The survivors are usually severely debilitated with spastic quadriplegia. Lesser degrees of cord damage at C5 to C6 may produce hand and forearm weakness with flexor weakness and wristdrop. Less commonly, the damage occurs at the C8 to T1 cord level, yielding extensor weakness with the fingers and hands ventriflexed. About 50 per cent of infants with so-called Erb's and Klumpke's pareses recover, usually by three to five months of age. Compression of the vertebral artery may occur, yielding secondary problems in the medullary area of the brain. A significant proportion of cerebral palsy cases of the past may relate to problems engendered by breech presentation with vaginal delivery. The late Dr. Nicholson Eastman of Johns Hopkins Hospital estimated that 24 per cent of cerebral palsy cases were associated with such problems.

Fractures of the femur, humerus, and clavicle are more common, as is bruising with secondary hyperbilirubinemia.[2] Tears of muscles may occur, and 20 per cent of instances of torticollis occur in babies who were in breech presentation. Another complication that may be secondary to breech vaginal delivery trauma is severance of the pituitary stalk with consequent hypopituitarism.[7] Vaginal breech delivery appears to be one of the most common causes of hypopituitarism, although it is realized that hypopituitarism is relatively rare.

MANAGEMENT, PROGNOSIS AND COUNSEL. In the prevention and management of breech presentation, three factors must be considered. First is prevention of the deformities and complications of vaginal delivery by moving the fetus into the vertex position long before the time of delivery by a method referred to as external cephalic version. Second is avoidance of the complications that relate to vaginal delivery of the breech fetus by accomplishing the delivery by cesarean section. Third is the management of any deformations and complications after delivery of the breech fetus.

External Cephalic Version. External cephalic version, the external manipulation of the fetus from the breech or transverse position into the vertex position, is a controversial procedure that is seldom taught as a part of obstetrics training today.[8] The major concern about the procedure is the potential risk to the fetus and mother versus the value of this measure. The procedural risk figures vary from zero to several per cent fetal mortality from such problems as early separation of the placenta, cord compression or prolapse, early rupture of membranes, and premature delivery.[8-10] In one study the overall complication rate was 4.4 per cent, which included fetal death in 0.9 per cent, premature labor in 1.2 per cent, and antepartum hemorrhage in 1.3 per cent. In addition, the attempt to accomplish external version is not always successful, and the fetus may revert back into the breech position before birth. Considering the other side of the question, successful external version limits the need for cesarean section and negates the risk of the deformations and complications involved in the vaginal delivery of a fetus in breech position.

The success rate for external version varies from about 30 to 98 per cent. The latter figure was obtained by Dr. Brooks Ranney of South Dakota, who accomplished 1240 external cephalic versions without a recognized complication for either the fetus or the pregnant woman.[11] Nearly two thirds of these fetuses reverted to an abnormal presentation and required repeat version. His recommendations include performing the version before 34 weeks of gestation. The mean age of version in his practice was 31 weeks. If one waits until after 34 to 35 weeks the size of the fetus in relation to the amount of amniotic fluid is such that successful and safe version is difficult. A second recommendation is that the maneuver be gentle. Neither analgesia nor anesthesia should be utilized. If gentle maneuvering does not work, the procedure should be stopped and tried again in a few days. External version should not be attempted if there are twins, if there is serious oligohydramnios, if the membranes have ruptured, if there is obvious placenta previa, or if the woman has diabetes mellitus, hypertension, or is Rh sensitized.

Utilizing external cephalic version, Dr. Ranney[11] reduced the frequency of breech presentation at birth from 4 per cent to 1 per cent and the frequency of prematurity related to breech or

Table 2–4. **FACTORS FAVORING CESAREAN SECTION DELIVERY OF THE FETUS IN BREECH PRESENTATION**

1. Scaphocephalic "breech head"
2. Hyperextended head
3. Contracted pelvis
4. Large baby, over 4.0 kg
5. Small baby, under 2.5 kg
6. Placenta previa
7. Maternal hypertension
8. Uterine dysfunction
9. Primigravida, especially if 35 years or older
10. Footling breech presentation
11. Previous pregnancy wastage

transverse presentation from 18 per cent to 3 per cent. The frequency of need for cesarean section was markedly reduced, and the perinatal mortality was reduced. It must be appreciated that these are the best results ever reported and that other observers have not had as great success with this maneuver. Though other physicians[12] have had results somewhat similar to those of Ranney, it is important to appreciate that most physicians are not experienced in performing the maneuver.

Cesarean Section. Given a fetus in breech presentation, the second line of prevention is to strive to forestall the potential complications of vaginal delivery by accomplishing a cesarean section when indicated.[1, 13-15] Table 2–4 lists some of the indications for a cesarean delivery.[1, 5, 12-14] As the concern for the complications of vaginal delivery of the breech fetus have increased in recent years, so also has the frequency of cesarean section for breech presentation. As previously mentioned, prolonged breech position in late fetal life tends to lead to a scaphocephalic "breech head," a deformity that enhances the risk of vaginal delivery. Sonography or roentgenography can be utilized to ascertain the extent of molding of the calvarium toward this elongated breech head. Its recognition may be used as an additional clue toward utilization of cesarean section rather than vaginal delivery. The scaphocephaly with prominent occipital shelf may create a serious problem in bringing the aftercoming head through the cervical opening. Such a head is more likely to become stuck during the second stage of labor. Attempts at extraction from below will enhance the risk of neurologic damage, such as brachial plexus palsy, cord tears, and/or temporary vertebral artery occlusion with potentially serious consequences.

MANAGEMENT OF DEFORMATIONS AND COMPLICATIONS. After birth the head shape as well as mandibular form gradually returns to normal with no management being indicated. If the hips

Table 2–5. **MALFORMATION DISORDERS THAT PREDISPOSE TO BREECH PRESENTATION**

Disorder	Breech Frequency	Explanation
Lower limb deficiency	60%	}————— Lack of leg thrust
Meningomyelocele in general	48%	
Meningomyelocele with leg paralysis	93%	
Anencephaly	excess	}————— Neurologic deficiency
Prader-Willi syndrome	50%	
Smith-Lemli-Opitz syndrome	40%	
Renal agenesis	50%	}————— Oligohydramnios with limited mobility
Severe polycystic kidneys	excess	
Urethral obstruction	excess	
Bicornuate uterus	excess	Crowding with limited mobility

are dislocated, a more rigorous management is indicated. The hydrocele of the testis is a benign lesion that rarely merits therapy. Tears of muscles may occur, and 20 per cent of instances of torticollis occur in babies who were in breech presentation.

DIFFERENTIAL DIAGNOSIS. The most important question about the infant with the breech deformation complex is whether an otherwise normal infant became caught in the breech position. If so, the prognosis, without birth complications, is usually excellent. If the infant was in the breech presentation *because* of a fetal problem, the prognosis relates predominantly to the basic diagnosis, with the addition of the secondary deformities due to breech presentation and/or the disruptive complications that may occur with vaginal delivery. The overall frequency of breech presentation in newborn babies with malformation problems is 23 per cent,[2] about eight times the general frequency. Such patients account for a sizeable proportion of the excess mortality of babies born in breech presentation. Certain types of malformation problems are notorious for failing to undergo normal version to a vertex presentation. The cause may be a structural defect, a neuromuscular defect, a renal defect resulting in oligohydramnios, or a problem of crowding. Table 2–5 lists some of the defects in which breech is a frequent consequence.[1, 5]

An elongated scaphocephalic head may also result from sagittal craniosynostosis. Usually palpation of the normally mobile sagittal suture is all that is required. Any doubt that might exist may generally be resolved by the follow-up, which shows progressive improvement toward normal form for the molded breech head. Roentgenograms are generally not indicated.

The shape of the head may yield a spuriously increased occipitofrontal head circumference, raising concern about hydrocephalus or macrocephaly. Generally this question can be readily resolved by simple examination of the head and sutures without further studies.

Dislocation of the hip may be engendered by a number of causes. When there is a basic problem in connective tissue that enhances the likelihood of mechanical dislocation, joints other than the hip are usually hypermobile. In the usual breech presentation patient who has dislocation of the hips, the joints are generally *less* mobile than usual, as a result of prolonged deficit in full range of movement.

Finally, the multiple consequences of prolonged breech presentation may be mistakenly interpreted as a multiple malformation disorder.

References

1. Dunn, P. M.: Maternal and fetal aetiological factors. 5th European Congress of Perinatal Medicine, Uppsala, Sweden, 1976, p. 76.
2. Dunn, P. M.: Breech delivery: Perinatal morbidity and mortality. 5th European Congress of Perinatal Medicine, Uppsala, Sweden, 1976, p. 54.
3. Kian, L. S.: The role of the placental site in the etiology of breech presentation. J. Obstet. Gynaecol. Br. Cwlth. 70:795, 1963.
4. Tompkins, P.: An inquiry into the causes of breech presentation. Am. J. Obstet. Gynecol. 51:595, 1946.
5. Haberkern, C., Smith, D. W., and Jones, K. L.: The "breech head" and its relevance. Am. J. Dis. Child. 133:154, 1979.
6. Cimmino, C. V., and Southworth, L. E.: Persistent hyperextension of the neck in breech and transverse lie: Indication for cesarean section. Am. J. Roentgenol. 125:447, 1975.
7. Rona, R. J., and Tanner, J. M.: Aetiology of idiopathic growth hormone deficiency in England and Wales. Arch. Dis. Child. 52:197, 1977.
8. Bradley-Watson, P. J.: The decreasing value of external cephalic version in modern obstetric practice. Am. J. Obstet. Gynecol. 123:237, 1975.
9. Friedlander, D.: External cephalic version in the management of breech presentation. A report of 706 patients treated by this method. Am. J. Obstet. Gynecol. 95:906, 1966.
10. Hibbard, L. T., and Schumann, W. R.: Prophylactic cephalic version in an obstetric practice. Am. J. Obstet. Gynecol. 116:511, 1973.
11. Ranney, B.: The gentle art of external cephalic version. Am. J. Obstet. Gynecol. 116:239, 1973.

12. Bock, J. E.: The influence of prophylactic external cephalic version on the incidence of breech delivery. Acta Obstet. Gynec. Scand. *48*:215, 1969.

13. Butler, N. R., and Bonham, D. G.: Perinatal mortality. The first report of the 1958 Perinatal Mortality Survey. London, E & S Livingstone, Ltd., 1963.

14. Hall, J. E., Kohl, S. G., O'Brien , F., and Ginsberg, M.: Breech presentation and perinatal mortality. A study of 6,044 cases. Am. J. Obstet. Gynecol. *91*:665, 1965.

15. Rovinsky, J. J., Miller, J. A., and Kaplan, S.: Management of breech presentation at term. Am. J. Obstet. Gynecol. *115*:497, 1973.

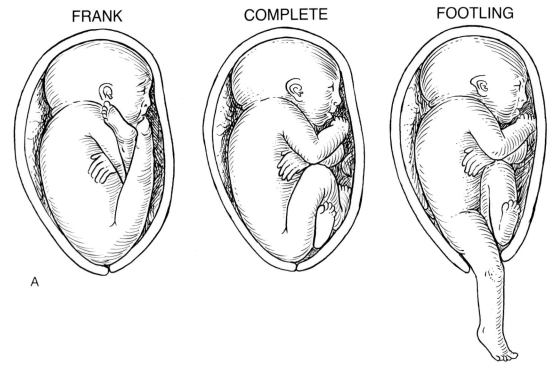

FRANK   COMPLETE   FOOTLING

A

Figure 2–33. Breech presentation deformation sequence. *A*, Types of breech presentation.

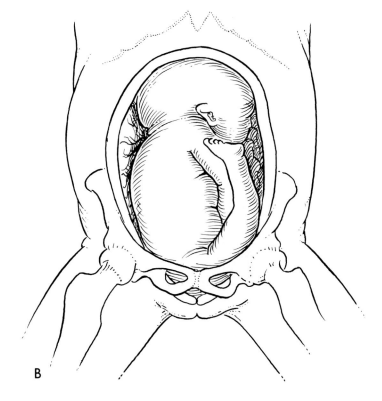

Figure 2–33 *Continued. B,* Frank breech presentation in utero in a term infant. (Adapted from in-utero roentgenograms and postnatal photos of Dunn, P. M.: Growth retardation of infant with congenital postural deformities. Acta Med. Auxol. 7:63, 1975.)

Illustration continued on following page

B

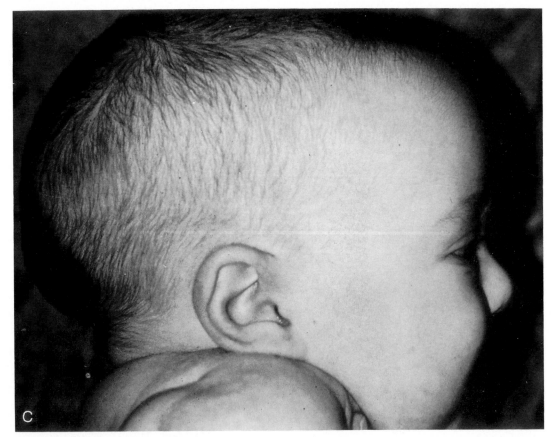

Figure 2–33 *Continued. C,* The scaphocephalic "breech head" with prominent occipital shelf in an infant. Note the tendency for the lower auricle to be uplifted by the upthrust of the shoulder in utero.

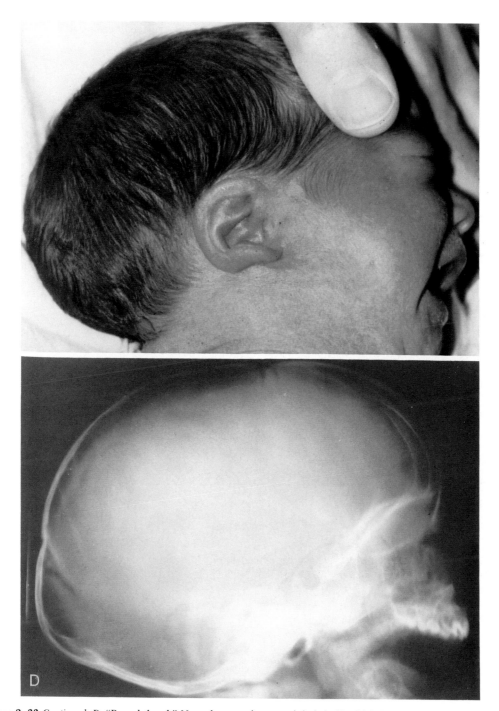

Figure 2–33 *Continued. D,* "Breech head." Note the prominent occipital shelf, which is evident on roentgenography.
Illustration continued on following page

Percentage of Deformations Related to Breech

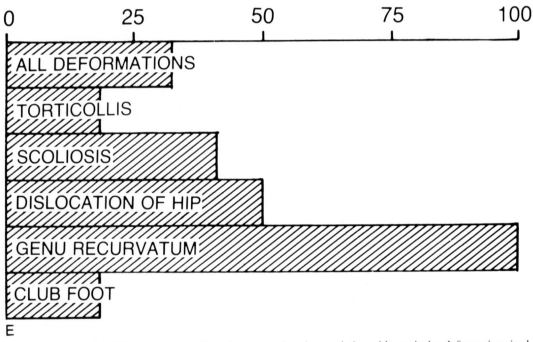

E

Figure 2–33 *Continued. E,* The percentage of breech presentations in association with particular deformations in the study of Dunn on some 6,000 newborn infants., (From Dunn, P. M.: Fifth European Congress of Perinatology, Uppsala, Sweden, 1976, p. 76.)

Figure 2–33 *Continued. F,* Extended knees and flexed thighs in a baby who had been in prolonged breech presentation and had bilaterally dislocated hips. Note the "breech head." *G,* Newborn baby who had been in the breech presentation in utero, showing flexed hips and extended knees in the "position of comfort" and great discomfort when the thighs are extended.
Illustration continued on following page

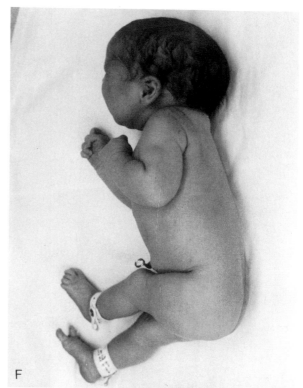

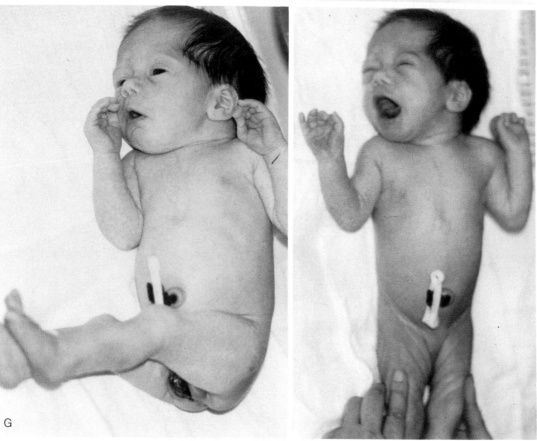

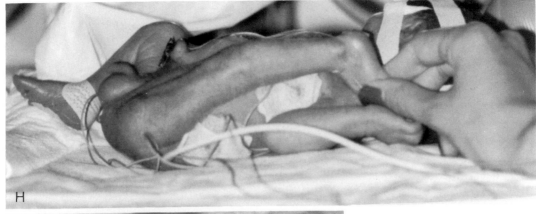

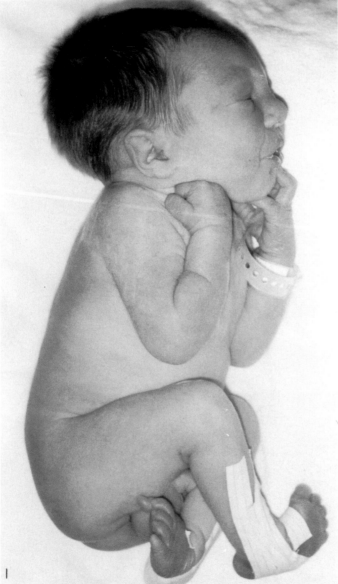

Figure 2–33 *Continued. H,* Prematurely born infant who had been in frank breech presentation shows genu recurvatum as a consequence. *I,* Infant who had been in frank presentation with flexed thighs and flexed lower legs. The equinovarus foot deformations, which are being treated by taping, are considered secondary to the complete breech presentation. Note the "breech head."

Figure 2–33 *Continued. J,* The edematous swelling on the labia majora and hemorrhagic edematous swelling of the labia minora and external vagina are secondary to prolonged constraint of this presenting part in the frank presentation. Look carefully for the ringlike zone around the buttocks and including the genitalia, which apparently represent the site of cervix indentation on the presenting part.

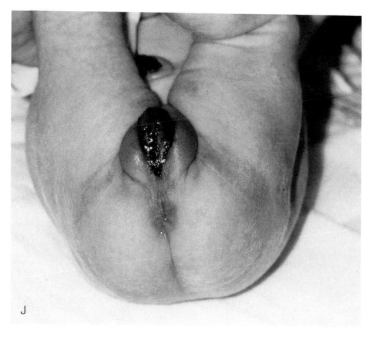

15. TRANSVERSE LIE DEFORMATION

COMMENT. Fortunately, transverse lie is rare, occurring once in about every 300 to 600 deliveries. It is more common in multiparous women. Most of the data regarding breech presentation are also applicable to transverse presentation. Hence only a few comments will be set forth.

GENESIS AND FEATURES. The lateral constraint may flatten the face, limit mandibular growth, cause a retroflexed head, and lead to scoliosis as well as other deformations (Fig. 2–34).

MANAGEMENT. Management is similar to that for breech position. Again, external cephalic version, a controversial procedure, merits consideration. However, it must be remembered that two common causes of transverse presentation, namely inlet contraction and placenta previa, would normally preclude vaginal delivery. Unresolved transverse presentation is usually an indication for cesarean section.

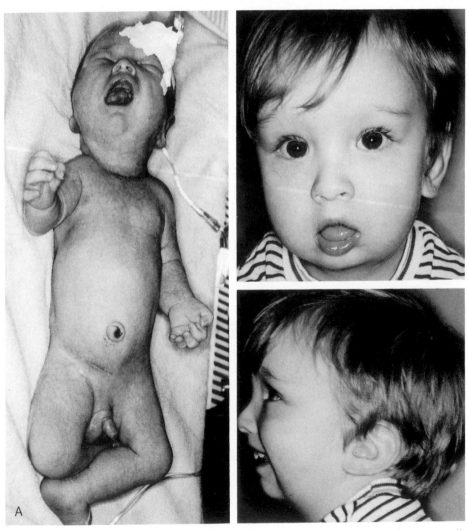

Figure 2–34. A, This infant was born at 36 weeks' gestation (left), having been in prolonged transverse lie since 17 weeks' gestation due to oligohydramnios resulting from slow leakage of amniotic fluid. By two and a half years of age (right) many of the facial deformations had resolved except for persistent micrognathia.

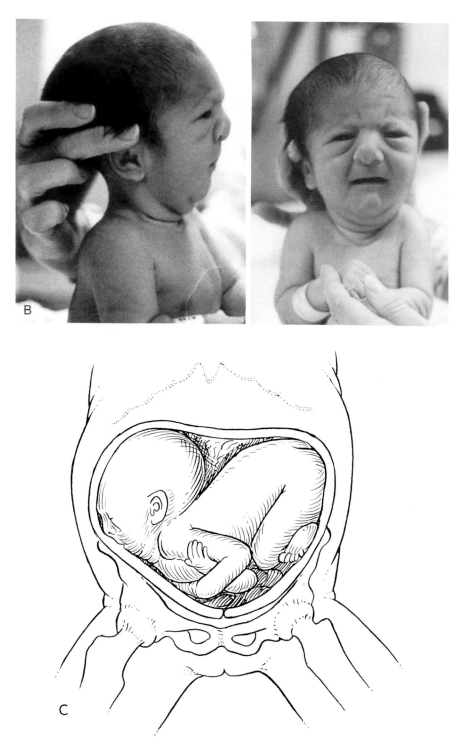

Figure 2–34 *Continued. B,* Flattening of the face with redundant "compression" skin in facies plus equinovarus foot deformities in an infant who had been in prolonged transverse presentation, apparently with the head retroflexed and the face forced against the wall of the uterus. The infant's appearance became progressively better and returned to normal form. (Courtesy of Dr. John Carey, from University of California Medical School, San Francisco.) *C,* Transverse presentation.

16. FACE AND BROW PRESENTATION DEFORMATION

GENESIS. In this presentation the face is the compressed presenting part, usually with extension of the head (Fig. 2–35). Face presentation occurs about once in 500 births, and persistent brow presentation is even less common.

FEATURES
Face Presentation. The growth of the mandible and nose may be restrained. The position of comfort for the baby after birth is often with the neck retroflexed. As a consequence of compression of the chin and neck region, with retroflexion there tend to be redundant folds of skin in the anterior upper neck.

Brow Presentation. The brow is unusually prominent, whereas the midface is less prominent than usual.

Face and brow presentation carry an increased risk of prematurity and of difficult labor. Compression of the neck against the pubic ramus during delivery can cause fracture of the trachea or the larynx. Cesarean section merits consideration, especially if the fetus is large or if the mother has a relatively small pelvis. Only anterior positions can be delivered vaginally because of the inability of the fetal neck to further extend in the posterior position.

MANAGEMENT AND PROGNOSIS.
Postnatally there tends to be catch-up of the restrained facial growth toward normal. The head gradually resumes a more normal posture, and the infant "grows into" the redundant skin that may be present on the anterior neck (face presentation). The parents need to be reassured that the infant is normal. There is generally no significant recurrence risk.

DIFFERENTIAL DIAGNOSIS
Face Presentation. The appearance of the face at birth may raise the question of a malformation problem such as Treacher-Collins syndrome or other craniofacial dysostosis. The malformation of the auricle and lower eyelid of Treacher-Collins syndrome tends to distinguish this disorder, as does a history of face presentation and the progressive postnatal improvement with the face presentation deformation.

Brow Presentation. The appearance of the face may suggest a craniofacial dysostosis problem such as Crouzon syndrome.

Anencephalic infants often manifest face presentations. Ninety per cent of deaths of babies born in face or brow presentation are infants with major malformation(s).

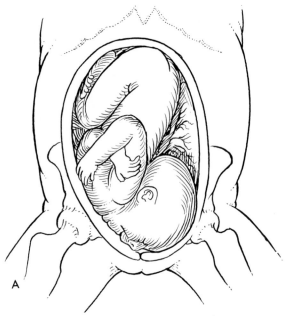

Figure 2–35. *A,* Face presentation.

References

1. von Reuss, A. R.: The Diseases of the Newborn. New York, William Wood and Co., 1921.
2. Butler, N. R., and Bonham, D. G.: Perinatal Mortal-
ity. The First Report of the 1958 British Perinatal Mortality Survey. London, E & S Livingstone Ltd., 1963.
3. Greenhill, J. P., and Friedman, E. A.: Biologic Principles and Modern Practice of Obstetrics. Philadelphia, W. B. Saunders Co., 1974.

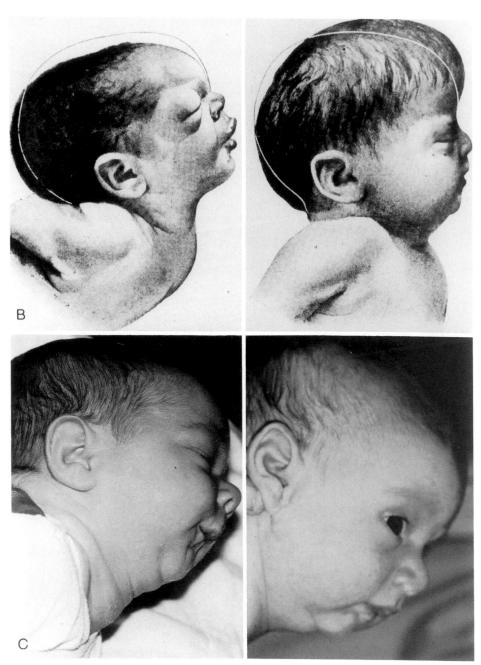

Figure 2–35 *Continued. B,* Examples of face and brow presentation; the white lines indicate the normal calvarial contour. (From von Ruess, A. R.: The Disease of the Newborn. New York, William Wood and Co., 1921.) *C,* Newborn infant of a small primigravida mother. The infant was in face presentation for at least the last two months of gestation, producing the extended head, the restricted nasal and mandibular growth, and the compressive overgrowth of skin in the anterior neck. By six weeks of age, the catch-up growth of the nose and mandible are evident, and the head is coming into a more normal alignment.

17. SMALL UTERINE CAVITY DEFORMATION

Malformed Uterus, Uterine Fibroid(s), Small Uterus

GENESIS. Several different problems may limit the size and/or shape of the uterus and thus enhance the likelihood of fetal deformation. Examples include a malformed uterus, most commonly bicornuate or unicornuate. It is estimated that 1 to 2 per cent of women have a malformation of the uterus and that the general risk of a deformation problem for the fetus in a malformed uterus is 30 per cent.[1] This would imply that three to six infants per 1000 have a deformation problem secondary to being gestated in a malformed uterus. Rarely, a large uterine fibroid may be the cause. Sometimes a small fibroma may enlarge rapidly under the influence of increased levels of estrogen during gestation. The small uterine cavity may result in miscarriage, stillbirth, fetal vascular disruption, or prematurity. It may also constrain the fetus and cause deformational problems.

FEATURES. All gradations of deformation of craniofacies, limbs, and thorax may occur, including overall constraint of fetal growth (Fig. 2–36). The constraint of thoracic growth may be sufficient to impair lung growth and maturation. Hence, some of these infants have respiratory distress at birth due to pulmonary hypoplasia.

MANAGEMENT, PROGNOSIS, AND COUNSEL. Insufficient uterine space for fetal growth should be considered as one possible explanation when a history of multiple miscarriages, stillbirths, prematurity, and/or serious deformation problems is obtained. Such findings may lead to the detection of a bicornuate uterus. Surgical improvement of the uterine size, if indicated and possible, may bring about a great improvement in the chances of rearing a normal fetus to a term birth. Large uterine fibroids may also merit consideration of surgical intervention.

If the infant born of a small uterine cavity has respiratory distress, all efforts should be utilized to maintain oxygenation. If the infant can survive the early neonatal period, the prognosis is usually good to excellent.

If dislocation of the hip is present, it obviously merits management. Recurrence risk counsel depends on the cause of the problem of limited uterine space for fetal growth. The risk could be quite high and might be appreciably reduced by attempts to improve the uterine space.

DIFFERENTIAL DIAGNOSIS. A history of multiple miscarriages, stillbirths, and "malformed offspring" may lead to a consideration of chromosomal studies of parents and offspring, in search of a balanced chromosomal transloction in one of the parents, with consequent unbalanced zygotes. Limited uterine space should also be considered in such situations, especially since it may be possible to improve the uterine situation by surgery in some instances. A careful assessment of infants born from a small uterine cavity who are considered "malformed" may indicate that they have multiple *deformations* rather than malformations.

Reference

1. Miller, M. E., Dunn, P. M., and Smith, D. W.: Uterine malformation and fetal deformation. J. Pediatr. *94*:387, 1979.

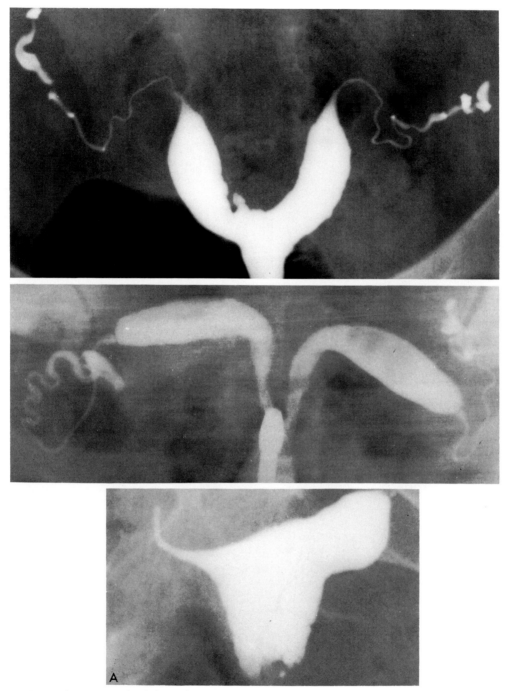

Figure 2–36. Small uterine cavity deformation. *A,* Three gradations of bicornuate uterus shown by hysterosalpingo-gram, each responsible for a deformational problem in the offspring.

Illustration continued on following page

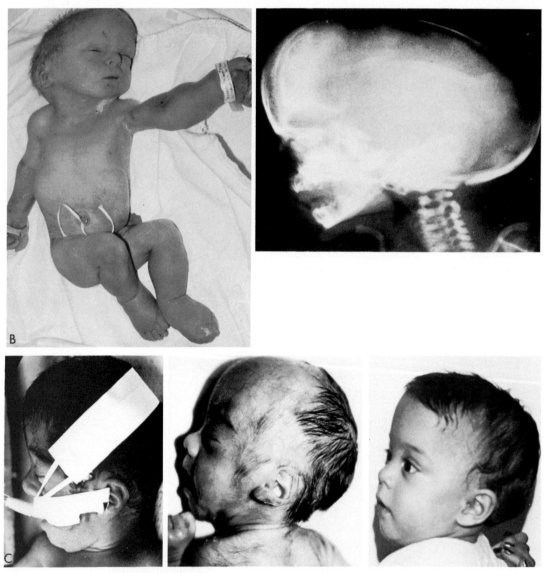

Figure 2–36 *Continued. B,* Severely deformed newborn infant gestated in a bicornuate uterus who died of respiratory insufficiency due to constraint-induced lung hypoplasia. The proximal constraint of limb has resulted in distal lymphedema, and the head has been molded out of alignment in such a manner as to give the impression of low placed ears. The mother had a history of five previous miscarriages. (From Miller, M. E., Dunn, P. M., and Smith, D. W.: Uterine malformation and fetal deformation. J. Pediatr. *94:*387,1979.) *C,* Prematurely born (34 weeks) infant with compressed craniofacies that initially had raised questions as to coronal craniostenosis. Within three weeks (middle) the face had grown forward and the question of craniostenosis was resolved. The right photo shows the infant at one year of age. (Courtesy of Dr. Kenneth Lyons Jones, University of California, San Diego. From Miller, M. E., Dunn, P. M., and Smith, D. W.: Uterine malformation and fetal deformation. J. Pediatr. *94:*387, 1979.)

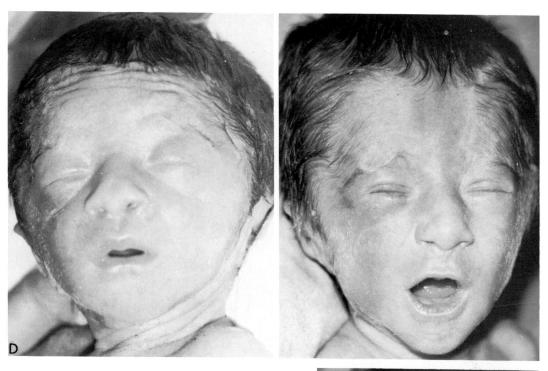

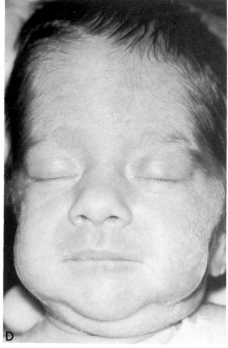

Figure 2–36 *Continued. D*, Prematurely born (34 weeks) infant gestated in a bicornuate uterus showing compressed facies with redundant skin. Follow-up at 48 hours and at 32 days shows the return toward normal form.

18. OLIGOHYDRAMNIOS SEQUENCE

GENESIS. The relative and absolute amount of amniotic fluid tends to decrease during the last trimester as the fetus is filling out the uterine cavity, as shown in Figure 2–37A. A serious deficiency of amniotic fluid will yield unusual uterine constraint. In early fetal life this deficiency may be secondary to amniotic rupture and may be accompanied by constrictive and disruptive bands and strands of amnion. The consequences of very early rupture with amniotic band disruptions can be horrendous and may include compressive consequences of early constraint, such as scoliosis and clubfeet, as well as vascular disruption leading to limb reduction and body wall defects. Such early cases are most commonly lethal and are found predominantly in spontaneous abortuses. Later rupture of the amnion may or may not be accompanied by amniotic bands. If later bands are present, they are usually limited to constrictive bands around various parts of one or more limbs. Chronic leakage of amniotic fluid, usually two to three or more weeks before delivery, is one cause of the oligohydramnios sequence (Figure 2–37B).

Oligohydramnios may occur with maternal hypertension, severe toxemia, placental insufficiency, and postmaturity, although the precise reason is unknown. It may also occur in one monozygotic twin because of placental vascular shunting. If one twin is transfusing the other, the donor tends to be hypovolemic with reduced renal blood flow, the presumed reason for the oligohydramnios.

Oligohydramnios may also be caused by a lack of adequate urine flow into the amniotic space because of a fetal malformation. The most common cause is renal agenesis, but it may also be due to polycystic kidneys or to obstructive uropathy. By the twentieth to twenty-fifth week of gestation, urine becomes a major constituent of amniotic fluid. Hence, oligohydramnios is predominantly a feature of these urinary tract malformations during the last half of gestation. Idiopathic oligohydramnios may also occur but is rare.

FEATURES. The features of the oligohydramnios sequence often include those of the breech deformation type, since about 50 per cent of these infants are in breech presentation at birth. As Smithells has aptly stated: "The fetus is in drydock and cannot maneuver for delivery."[2]

Craniofacial. The head usually looks as though a silk stocking had been pulled down over it, causing a flattened nose and flattened or "accordioned" external ears.

Limbs. The hands and feet—especially the feet— tend to be in aberrant position, often with stiffness of the joints, which have been limited in their mobility. The hips may be dislocated.

Thorax and Lungs. Thoracic growth is restrained, and the full growth and maturation of the lung is thwarted.[1] The lungs often do not progress beyond a four to five month level of development and hence may be hypoplastic, lacking in surfactant, and incapable of aerobic expansion and/or oxygen exchange. This respiratory insufficiency is the most common cause of demise in the immediate postnatal period. Not uncommonly, attempts to resuscitate the newborn baby lead to pneumothorax, a frequent complication in the baby with respiratory insufficiency due to oligohydramnios.

Skin. The skin tends to be redundant, presumably the result of overgrowth related to external constraint. This gives rise to accentuated inner canthal and infraorbital skin folds, which contribute to the "Potter" facies and sometimes yield the impression of a webbed neck.

Other. Concretions of amnion cells may build up on the relatively dry surface of the placenta, a feature termed *amnion nodosa*. The umbilical cord is usually short.[3]

MANAGEMENT, PROGNOSIS, AND COUNSEL. If the oligohydramnios is due to renal agenesis or another type of severe renal problem, attempts to oxygenate the neonate artificially are of little or no value. However, if the deficit of amniotic fluid is due to chronic leakage of amniotic fluid, then every attempt toward oxygenation should be pursued, since the renal function is normal. If such an infant survives, there is usually catch-up growth with a restitution toward normal form. The recurrence risk relates to the basic problem that gave rise to the oligohydramnios. Thus, with chronic leakage of fluid the recurrence risk would be very low. With defects such as obstructive uropathy or renal agenesis the risk may be higher. Renal agenesis may recur and may be associated with renal anomalies in first degree relatives.[4] With infantile polycystic kidney disease, the risk may be as high as 25 per cent (autosomal recessive). Prenatal diagnosis should be offered for subsequent pregnancies when oligohydramnios is due to a fetal malformation problem.

DIFFERENTIAL DIAGNOSIS. See *Genesis*.

References

1. Thomas, I. T., and Smith, D. W.: Oligohydramnios, cause of the non-renal features of Potter's syndrome,

including pulmonary hypoplasia. J. Pediatr. *84*:811, 1974.

2. Scott, J. S.: The volume and circulation of the liquor amnii: Clinical observations. Proc. Roy. Soc. Med. *59*:1128, 1966.
3. Miller, M. E., Higginbottom, M. C., and Smith, D. W.: Short umbilical cord: Its origin and relevance. Pediatrics *67*:5, 1981.
4. Morse, R. P., Rawnsley, B. E., Crow, H. C., Marin-Padilla, M., and Graham, J. M., Jr.: Bilateral renal agenesis in three consecutive siblings. Prenatal Diagnosis, *7*:573, 1987.

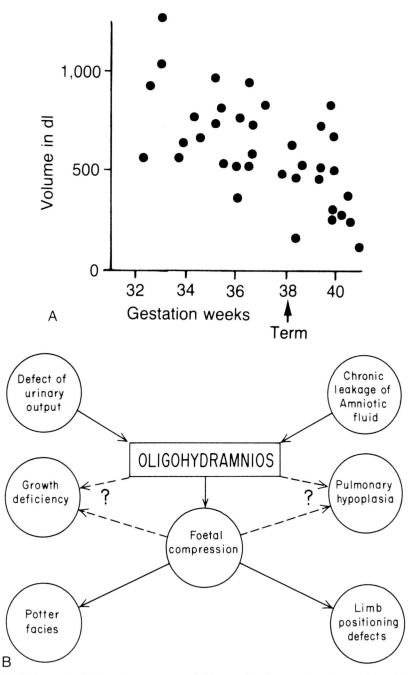

Figure 2–37. Oligohydramnios deformation sequence. *A*, Progressive decrease in volume of amniotic fluid during the last trimester. *B*, Origins and impact of oligohydramnios on the fetus.

Illustration continued on following page

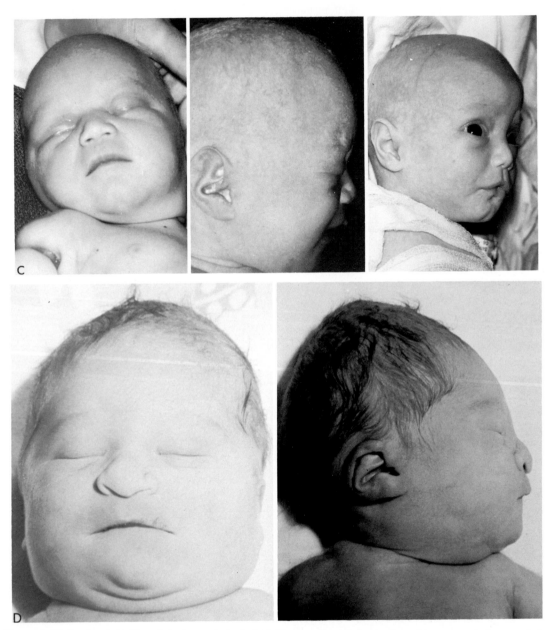

Figure 2–37 *Continued. C,* Chronic leakage of amniotic fluid since 15 weeks' gestation with one amniotic constrictive band on the upper arm. Oligohydramnios sequence included flattened nose, auricle, and loose skin. Oxygenation was maintained for transient respiratory insufficiency, and the infant returned toward normal form by six weeks (right). *D,* Compressed face, redundant skin, and accordion ear of a newborn infant with severe oligohydramnios secondary to renal agenesis.

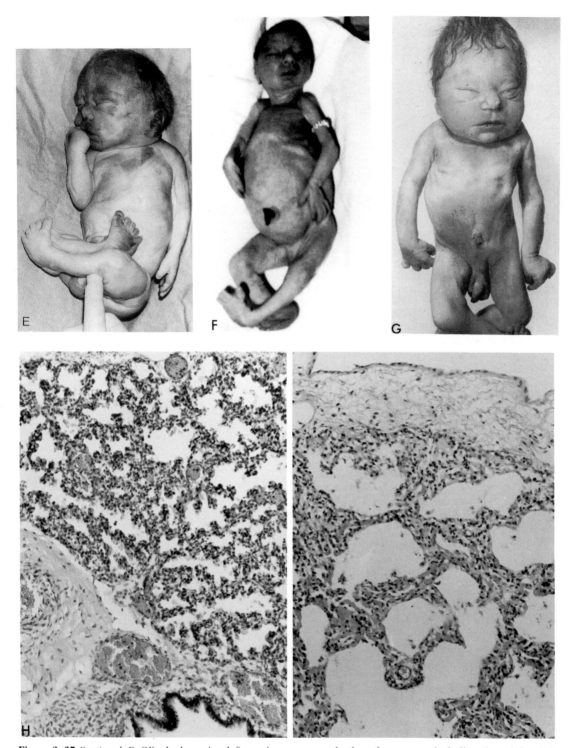

Figure 2–37 *Continued. E*, Oligohydramnios deformation sequence plus breech sequence, including "breech head" in an infant with chronic leakage of amniotic fluid for six weeks prior to delivery. Note the redundant skin. *F*, Oligohydramnios sequence with severe deficit of thoracic growth and limb deformation in an infant with massive polycystic kidneys that have distended the abdomen. *G*, Renal agenesis with severe oligohydramnios. Note the effects not only on the limbs but also on the thoracic cage. *H*, Lung hypoplasia secondary to severe oligohydramnios yielding non-expansile lung with limited aerobic exchange, in contrast to normal lung (right). (From Thomas, I. T., and Smith, D. W.: Oligohydramnios, cause of the non-renal features of Potter's syndrome. J. Pediatr. *84*:811, 1974.)

19. FETAL AKINESIA SEQUENCE

GENESIS. Fetal movement is essential to normal morphogenesis. To provide appropriate care and counseling, it is most important to distinguish extrinsic factors that limit fetal movement (e.g., oligohydramnios or fetal crowding) from intrinsic factors due to neuromuscular abnormalities. Both types of problems can prevent normal version and lead to abnormalities of fetal presentation. Intrinsic neuromuscular abnormalities may prevent the fetus from undergoing normal version, hence the association between breech presentation and fetal abnormalities.[1]

Fetal immobilization during late gestation can give rise to transient joint limitation in normal newborns. Movement is an important factor in normal joint morphogenesis. Joints develop secondarily within the condensed mesenchyme of the developing bones, and chronic lack of movement tends to give rise to joint contractures.[2, 3] Moessinger demonstrated that rat fetuses paralyzed by daily transuterine injections of curare from day 18 of gestation until day 21 (term) demonstrated a pattern of abnormalities that he termed fetal akinesia deformation sequence.[3] The consequences of fetal akinesia during late gestation can include multiple joint contractures, micrognathia, polyhydramnios, pulmonary hypoplasia, fetal growth retardation, and short umbilical cord (Figs. 2–38 and 2–39). This phenotype is not specific but instead represents an etiologically heterogeneous deformation sequence that can result from a variety of congenital neuropathies or myopathies that must be distinguished from extrinsic fetal immobilization.

One dramatic human example was an infant born with multiple joint contractures (termed *arthrogryposis*) whose mother had received tubocurarine for 19 days in early pregnancy for the treatment of tetanus.[4] There is evidence in both experimental animals and humans that fetal akinesia due to a variety of causes can lead to multiple joint contractures and the other manifestations of fetal akinesia sequence.[2–6]

The fetal akinesia phenotype occurs in type 1 Pena-Shokeir syndrome, an autosomal recessive disorder[7–9] and also in a number of other genetic fetal malformation syndromes.[10] Maternal myotonic dystrophy can interact with a genetically affected fetus to produce this phenotype[11] (Fig. 2–39*A*), and similar effects have been noted in infants born to mothers with myasthenia gravis due to transplacental transfer of immunoglobulins that are thought to create a neuromuscular blockade in the fetus[12] (Fig. 2–39*B* and *C*). The severity of fetal akinesia sequence may depend on the timing, duration, and degree of fetal akinesia (Fig. 2–39*D*).

Duration of fetal akinesia may be determined through an analysis of the individual features. Prolonged immobilization limits bone growth, affecting subperiosteal growth in bone breadth much more severely than linear growth. This leads to the development of thin bones that may be susceptible to fractures. The size of a muscle relates to the magnitude and frequency of forces, and with diminished function, muscles tend to atrophy. Thus prolonged fetal akinesia results in low birth weight. Absence of flexion creases implies that the joint has never functioned; since most joints function by the early second trimester, this implies early cessation of fetal movement. Polyhydramnios is a relatively late manifestation of the fetal akinesia sequence.[10] It is usually associated with micrognathia due to diminished fetal swallowing.

Fetal lung movements are necessary for normal pulmonary growth and maturation. The importance of fetal respiratory movements in normal lung morphogenesis was highlighted by a case report describing an infant with pulmonary hypoplasia due to phrenic nerve agenesis and diaphragmatic amyoplasia.[13] In an experimental fetal rabbit model, destruction of the fetal cervical cord in the C4–C6 region caused complete atrophy of the diaphragm, in addition to cutting off motor pathways from the respiratory center. Higher lesions at C1–C3 preserved the phrenic nerve supply and hence allowed normal diaphragmatic growth but prevented any coordinated fetal respiratory activity. Either operation performed at 23 days gestation, during the late pseudoglandular phase of lung development, resulted in severe lung hypoplasia.[14] Thus with severe fetal akinesia inhibiting fetal swallowing and fetal lung movements, the fetus is born with micrognathia, polyhydramnios, and respiratory insufficiency from pulmonary hypoplasia.

The association of a shortened umbilical cord implies fetal akinesia that began during or prior to midgestation. Umbilical cord growth is influenced by tensile forces and depends on both fetal motion and the amount of space available for fetal movement.[15] This has been demonstrated in both the human and the rat.[15, 16]

Since oligohydramnios can severely limit fetal movement during the last half of gestation, there may be overlap between the oligohydramnios sequence and the fetal akinesia sequence. Compression of skin in the oligohydramnios sequence leads to redundancy, whereas fetal akinesia leads to thin, tight skin with few flexion creases. Deformations associated with polyhydramnios usually imply an intrinsic neuromuscular abnormality.

FEATURES. The features of the fetal akinesia sequence often include those of the breech presentation deformation type. These features are also characteristic of type 1 Pena-Shokeir syndrome,[15] an autosomal recessive disorder that is estimated to occur in 1 in 12,000 births (probably reflecting etiologic heterogeneity).

Growth. There is prenatal onset growth deficiency with associated polyhydramnios leading to prematurity in some instances.

Brain and Neuromuscular. A variety of congenital neuropathies and myopathies may limit fetal movement.[17]

Craniofacial. Micrognathia with small mouth, depressed tip of the nose, and limited extension of the head occur. The eyes appear wide-set, and the ears appear low-set.

Limbs. The hands, and especially the feet, tend to be in aberrant position, leading to camptodactyly and equinovarus foot deformations. The long bones may be thin with decreased muscular bulk.

Thorax and Lungs. There is pulmonary hypoplasia with low lung weight or a low lung/body weight ratio at autopsy. Deficient alveolarization with decreased surfactant may lead to fetal respiratory insufficiency in the perinatal period. The ribs may appear thin.

Skin. The skin appears thin and tight, with deficient or absent flexion creases. Webbing of skin across a joint may occur with early limitations of movement.

Other. The umbilical cord is short. Polyhydramnios may be present, as may occasional cryptorchidism or hip dislocation.

MANAGEMENT, PROGNOSIS, AND COUNSEL.

If the akinesia is due to a neuropathy or myopathy, attempts to oxygenate the neonate may be unsuccessful due to underlying pulmonary hypoplasia. If late gestational constraint has immobilized the fetus, then vigorous orthopedic management and physical therapy are merited, and there is a good prognosis. The recurrence risk relates to the basic problem that gave rise to the akinesia. With congenital neuropathies and myopathies, the recurrence risk may be quite high.[17]

DIFFERENTIAL DIAGNOSIS. See *Genesis*.

References

1. Braun, F. H. T., Jones, K. L., and Smith, D. W.: Breech presentation as an indication of fetal abnormality. J. Pediatr. 86:419, 1975.
2. Drachman, D. B., and Coulombre, A. J.: Experimental clubfoot and arthrogryposis multiplex congenita. Lancet 2:523, 1962.
3. Moessinger, A. C.: Fetal akinesia sequence: An animal model. Pediatrics 72:857, 1983.
4. Jago, R. H.: Arthrogryposis following treatment of maternal tetanus with muscle relaxants. Arch. Dis. Child. 45:277, 1970.
5. Hall, J. G., and Reed, S. D.: Teratogens associated with congenital contractures in humans and in animals. Teratology 25:173, 1982.
6. Swinyard, C. A.: Concept of multiple congenital contractures (arthrogryposis) in man and animals. Teratology 25:247, 1982.
7. Pena, S. D. J., and Shokeir, M. H. K.: Syndrome of camptodactyly, multiple ankyloses, facial anomalies, and pulmonary hypoplasia: A lethal condition. J. Pediatr. 85:373, 1974.
8. Punnett, H. H., Kistenmacher, M. L., Valdes-Dpena, M., et al.: Syndrome of ankylosis, facial anomalies and pulmonary hypoplasia. J. Pediatr. 85:375, 1984.
9. Williams, R. S., and Holmes, L. B.: The syndrome of multiple ankyloses and facial anomalies, a neuropathologic analysis. Acta Neuropathol. 50:175, 1980.
10. Morse, R. P., Rawnsley, B. E., Sargent, S. K., and Graham, J. M., Jr.: Prenatal diagnosis of a new syndrome: Holoprosencephaly with hypokinesia. Prenatal Diagnosis, 7:631, 1987.
11. Bell, D. B., and Smith, D. W.: Myotonic dystrophy in the neonate. J. Pediatr. 81:83, 1972.
12. Holmes, L. B., Driscoll, S. G., and Bradley, W. G.: Contractures in an infant of a mother with myasthenia gravis. J. Pediatr. 96:1067, 1980.
13. Goldstein, J. D., and Reid, L. M.: Pulmonary hypoplasia resulting from phrenic nerve agenesis. J. Pediatr. 97:282, 1980.
14. Wigglesworth, J. S., and Desai, R.: Effects on lung growth of cervical cord section in the rabbit fetus. Early Human Devel. 3:51, 1979.
15. Miller, M. E., Higginbottom, M. C., and Smith, D. W.: Short umbilical cords: Its origin and relevance. Pediatrics 67:5, 1981.
16. Moessinger, A. C., Blanc, W. A., Marone, P. A., et al.: Umbilical cord length as an index of fetal activity: Experimental study and clinical implications. Pediatr. Res. 16:109, 1982.
17. Hall, J. G.: Invited editorial comment: Analysis of Pena-Shokeir phenotype. Am. J. Med. Genet. 25:99, 1986.

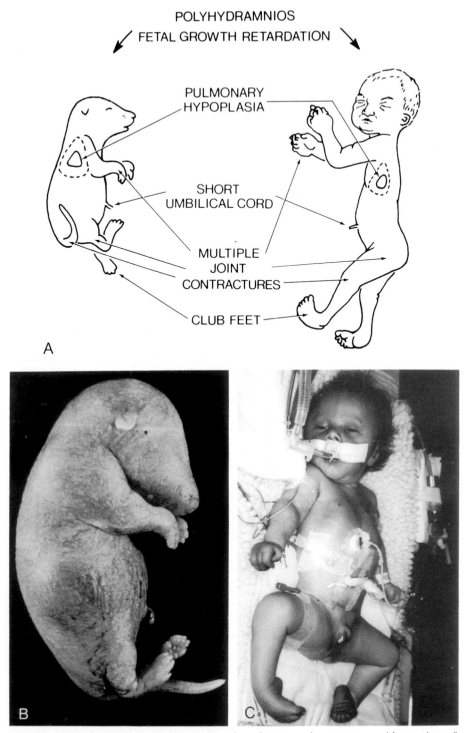

Figure 2–38. *A,* The fetal akinesia deformation sequence is a phenotype that can occur with a variety of congenital neuropathies and myopathies (right). It has been modeled experimentally in rat fetuses paralyzed by daily transuterine injections of curare from day 18 of gestation until term (day 21). *B,* An affected rat fetus at term reveals joint contractures and thin, tight skin with few flexion creases. *C,* The newborn with Type I Pena-Shokeir syndrome was born with polyhydramnios, lethal pulmonary hypoplasia, and joint contractures. Attempts to diagnose a subsequent recurrence during the second trimester were unsuccessful, but polyhydramnios and limited fetal movement were evident during the third trimester. (*A* and *B* from Moessinger, A. C.: Fetal akinesia deformation sequence: An animal model. Pediatrics 72:857, 1983. Reproduced by permission of Pediatrics.)

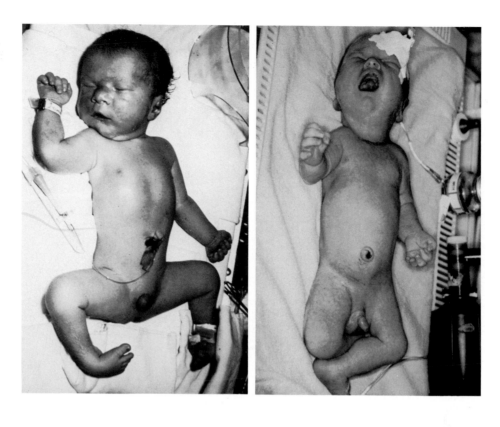

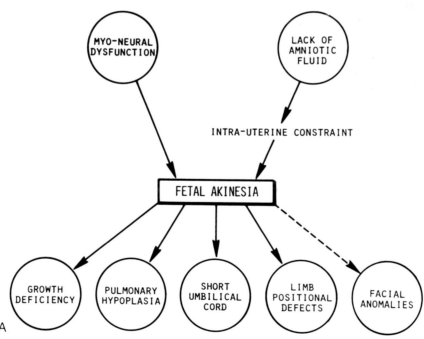

A

Figure 2–39. *A*, The diagram at the bottom demonstrates the etiologically heterogeneous phenotype that results from fetal akinesia. The infant at the top left was born with myotonic dystrophy to a mother with the same condition. He had multiple joint contractures with thin bones and respiratory insufficiency. The infant at the top right was severely constrained from 17 weeks' gestation until term due to leaking amniotic fluid. Vigorous orthopedic management and physical therapy led to partial improvement.

Illustration continued on following page

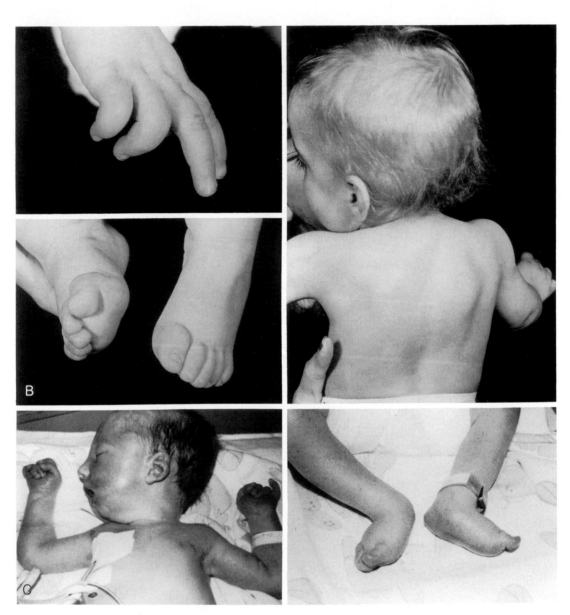

Figure 2–39 *Continued. B,* This infant was born to a mother with myasthenia gravis. Both she and a subsequent sibling were born with hypotonia, multiple joint contractures, and severe scoliosis. (Courtesy of Dr. Mark Stephan, Tacoma, WA.) *C,* This infant was born with severe hypotonia and equinovarus foot deformities. (From Holmes et al. Contractures in an infant of a mother with myasthenia gravis. J. Pediatr. *96*:1067, 1980.)

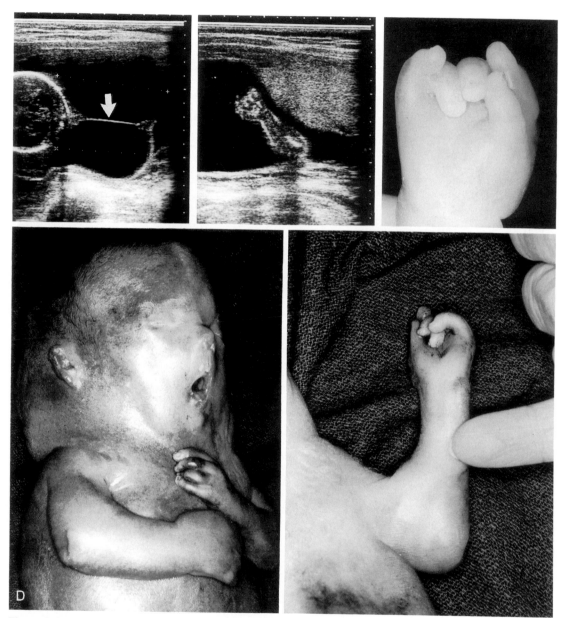

Figure 2–39 *Continued. D,* This fetus was recognized by prenatal ultrasound as having virtually no fetal movement and a large nuchal cystic hygroma with a midline septation (arrow, top left). The hands were observed to be clenched by ultrasound, with no finger creases on examination (top right). Amniocentesis revealed a 46,XX karyotype, and multiple pterygia were noted postnatally, as illustrated by the shoulder girdle pterygium (lower right). This illustrates the severe consequences of prolonged fetal akinesia in a fetus with lethal multiple pterygium syndrome and nuchal cystic hygroma. Muscle pathology demonstrated neurogenic atrophy.

20. EXTRAUTERINE PREGNANCY

GENESIS, FEATURES, PROGNOSIS. In rare instances fertilization of the ovum may take place outside the fallopian tube, and the zygote may then implant outside the uterus (Fig. 2–40). When this occurs the conceptus seldom survives. Oligohydramnios is frequent.[1] If survival does occur, there is likely to be severe constraint of fetal development.

The incidence of abdominal pregnancy is one in 50,820 deliveries, and survival is greatly improved if the amniotic sac remains intact.[2] The overall mortality rate is 75 to 95 per cent,[3] with death usually resulting from pulmonary hypoplasia associated from oligohydramnios and prolonged fetal thoracic compression.[4]

References

1. Scott, J. S.: The volume and circulation of the liquor amnii. Clinical observations. Proc. Roy. Soc. Med. *59*:1128, 1966.
2. Tan, K. L., Goon, S. M., and Wee, J. H.: The pediatric aspects of advanced abdominal pregnancy. J. Obstet. Gynaec. Br. Commonwealth *76*:1021, 1969.
3. Delke, I., Veridanio, N. P., Tancer, M. L.: Abdominal pregnancy: Review of current management and addition of ten cases. Obstet. Gynecol. *60*:200, 1982.
4. Bell, J. B., Gerdes, J. S., Bhutani, V. K., Wilmott, R. W.: A chronic lung disorder following abdominal pregnancy. Am. J. Dis. Child. *141*:1111, 1987.

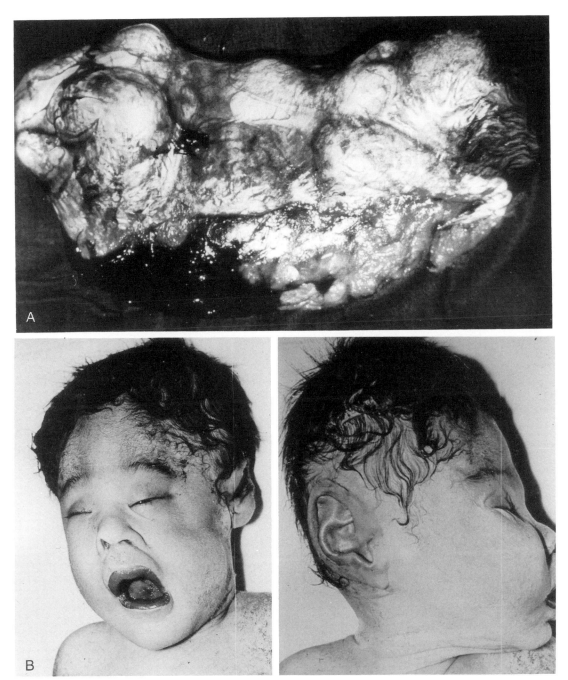

Figure 2–40. *A,* Extrauterine pregnancy showing intact amniotic sac that contains no amniotic fluid and encases the compressed fetus. (Courtesy of Dr. Scott, Department of Obstetrics and Gynecology, Leeds, England.) *B,* This infant was delivered abdominally from an extrauterine location behind the uterus. Note the marked distortion of the face and compressive overgrowth of the right ear. Respiratory insufficiency associated wtih oligohydramnios led to death shortly after birth. (Courtesy of Dr. Will Cochran of Beth Israel Hospital and Harvard Medical School, Boston.)

21. EARLY CONSTRAINT DEFECTS

Constraint that occurs during the latter period of gestation usually causes molded deformations with good prospects for spontaneous or assisted return to normal form. However, constraint that occurs in early morphogenesis can have more severe and lasting impacts on form (Fig. 2–41). The types of defects that can be produced by constraint within the first trimester fall into three categories, as summarized in Table 2–6.

All three types of defects were experimentally produced by Poswillo[1] by early amniotic sac puncture in rat embryos of 15½ days' gestation. At that time the rat embryo is at about the same stage as the human is at six to seven weeks of gestation. The mesenchymal condensations of the limb bones have occurred, but the fingers are not fully separated. The lip is fused, but the palatal shelves have yet to close. Following puncture of the amnion, the animals were found to be compressed in a cephalocaudal fashion with the developing mandible thrust against the sternum and the limbs in various stages of compression. Table 2–7 summarizes the frequency of the three types of defects observed in the 32 animals so treated.[1] There were no defects in the control animals. All treated animals showed a small jaw, caused by compression of the mandible against the sternum. In all but one fetus this had caused the tongue to be maintained between the palatal shelves thereby preventing closure of the palatal shelves. The failure of full separation of the fingers (syndactyly) was also interpreted as incomplete morphogenesis secondary to compression. The loss of the radius, the femur, and major limb parts, which must have been normally present at the time of the induced compression, was interpreted as the result of focal hemorrhage and necrosis. Kennedy and Persaud have shown that the amnion puncture leads to edema and hemorrhage with tissue damage and resorption.[2] Webster has demonstrated that a broad variety of uterine manipulations in pregnant mice at this early stage of gestation can result in hemorrhagic disruption of various fetal structures.[3]

We are only beginning to appreciate comparable defects in man as presumed consequences of early compression in utero. Among the patients with early rupture of the amnion who have amniotic bands, we have observed talipes deformations, syndactyly, and limb reductions of a type that could not be readily explained by amniotic band constrictions.[4, 5] Bands were also present in 19 per cent of the rats in Poswillo's study.[1] Among early amnion rupture cases in the human, we have observed scoliosis and other deformations.[4, 5]

We have also observed instances of the Robin malformation sequence, formerly termed Pierre Robin syndrome, in which the total findings were compatible with a constraint causation for the early micrognathia and obstruction of palatine closure by the tongue as cause of a secondary posterior cleft palate. Poswillo[1] found that 29 per cent of rat fetuses with the Robin sequence defects induced by oligohydramnios compression also had limb defects, most commonly deformational in type. Dunn[6] states that half of his human patients with Robin sequence defects had deformations, especially of the limb. Hanson and Smith[7] report that 11 per cent of their patients in whom Robin sequence was part of a known syndrome also had limb defects.

We have observed early limb compressive effects of all three types (Table 2–6) in individuals who had been reared in a constrictive bicornuate uterus or a uterus with large fibroids.[4, 5] Matsunaga and Shiota[8] also have recognized early spatial limitation as a factor in constraint-induced malformation. They found that 11.6 per cent of 43 embryos

Table 2–6. TYPES OF DEFECTS PRODUCED IN EARLY GESTATION BY CONSTRAINT

1. *Molded deformations:* Similar to those produced in late fetal life, but often more severe and difficult to return to normal form because of early onset.
2. *Incomplete morphogenesis:* The constraint may limit or prevent full completion of a normal stage in morphogenesis.
3. *Disruption of morphogenesis:* The constraint may cause edema, hemorrhage, and focal necrosis with loss of previously formed tissue.

Table 2–7. DEFECTS FOUND BY POSWILLO IN 32 RAT FETUSES FOLLOWING OLIGOHYDRAMNIOS COMPRESSION AT 15½ DAYS (similar to 42–45 days in human)

1. Molded deformations	100%
a. Micrognathia	100%
b. Talipes	5%
2. Incomplete morphogenesis	97%
a. Failure of palatal closure	97%
b. Syndactyly	9%
3. Disruption of morphogenesis	12%
a. Absent radius, femur	6%
b. Phocomelia	6%

(From Poswillo, D.: Observations of fetal posture and causal mechanisms of congenital deformity of the palate, mandible and limbs. J. Dent. Res. *45*(3):583, 1966.)

and fetuses recovered from ectopic tubal pregnancies had structural defects, as did 6.2 per cent of 97 fetuses from myomatous pregnancies, in contrast to 3.3 per cent structural defects among 3474 normally implanted therapeutic abortuses from non-myomatous uteri. Two of the five fetuses with structural defects who were reared in the fallopian tube had amelia.[8]

References

1. Poswillo, D.: Observations of fetal posture and causal mechanisms of congenital deformity of the palate, mandible and limbs. J. Dent. Res. *45*(3):583, 1966.
2. Kennedy, L. A., and Persaud, T. V. N.: Pathogenesis of developmental defects induced in the rat by amniotic sac puncture. Acta Anat. (Basel) *97*:23, 1977.
3. Webster, W. S., Lipson, A. H., and Brown-Woodman, P. D. C.: Uterine trauma and limb defects. Teratology *35*:253, 1987.
4. Graham, J. M., Jr.: The association between limb anomalies and spatially restricting uterine environments. Progr. Clin. Biol. Res. *163C*:99, 1985.
5. Graham, J. M., Jr., Miller, M. E., Stephan, M. J., and Smith, D. W.: Limb reduction anomalies and early in-utero limb compression. J. Pediatr. *96*:1052, 1980.
6. Dunn, P. M.: The influence of the intrauterine environment in the causation of congenital postural deformities, with special reference to congenital dislocation of the hip. MD thesis, University of Cambridge, 1969.
7. Hanson, J. W., and Smith, D. W.: U-shaped palatal defect in the Robin anomalad: Developmental and clinical relevance. J. Pediatr. *87*:30, 1975.
8. Matsunaga, E., and Shiota, K.: Ectopic pregnancy and myoma uteri: Teratogenic effects and maternal characteristics. Teratology, *21*:61, 1980.

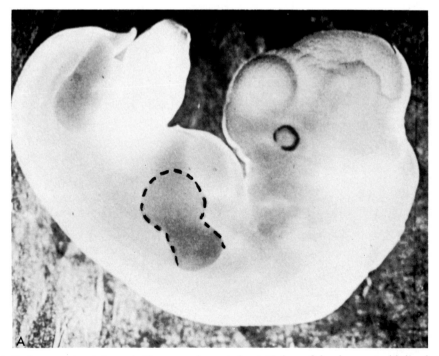

Figure 2–41. Early constraint defects. *A,* Human embryo at about 42 days of development with hand plate formed (outlined) but no separation of the finger rays. It is around this era that constraint of the developing limb has been shown in animal studies to cause edema, hemorrhage, and resorptive necrosis with loss of previously normal tissues. The process of separation of the digits may also be impaired, yielding syndactyly.

Illustration continued on following page

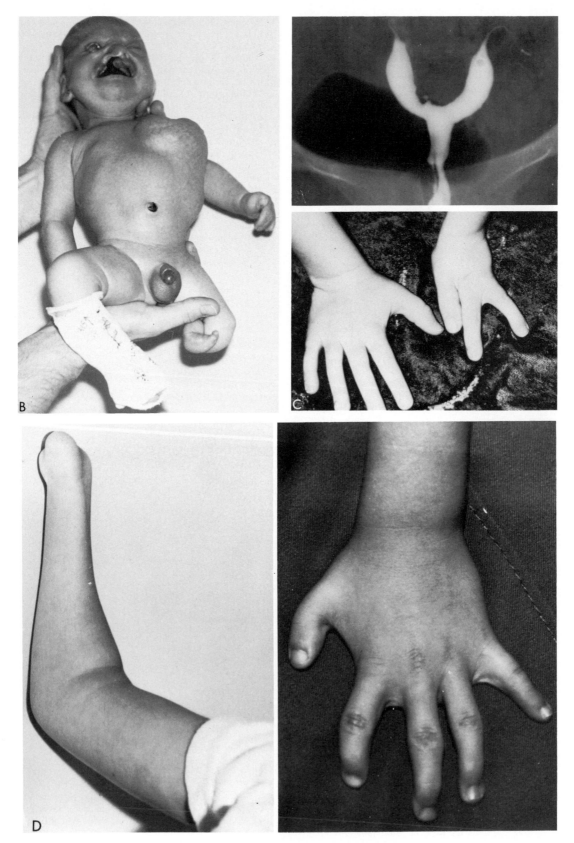

Figure 2–41 *Continued. See legend on opposite page*

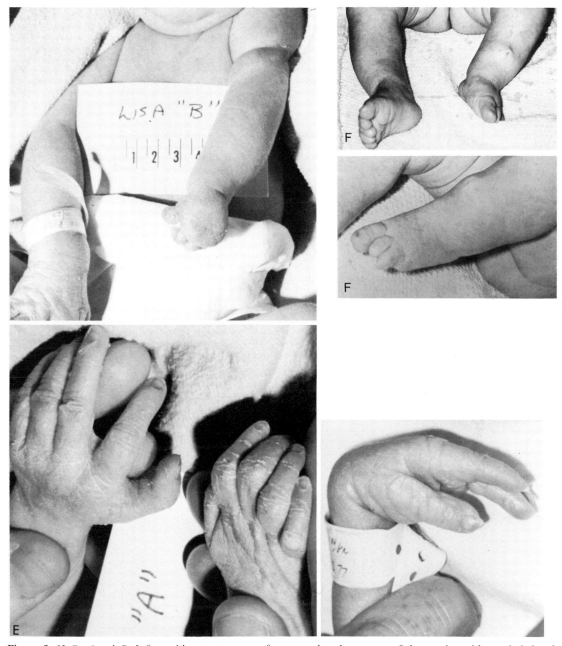

Figure 2–41 *Continued. B,* Infant with consequences of presumed early rupture of the amnion with amniotic band disruption of right facies including eye, disruption of left thoracic cage, and band constriction on left thumb. In addition, there is partial limb reduction of the left lower limb and failure of separation of the left second and third fingers, presumed effects of the early constraint and vascular disruption at the time of amnion rupture. *C,* Unilateral oligodactyly in a child reared in the above bicornuate uterus. *D,* Lack of distal arm and contralateral hypoplasia of thumb and mild second to third finger syndactyly in a child reared in a bicornuate uterus. *E* Monozygotic, monoamniotic twins with early rupture of amnion leading to amniotic band with distal arm and hand hypoplasia in twin B (above), whereas twin A (below) has a unilateral radial nerve palsy with small arm on the affected side. This neurologic deficit was interpreted as the consequence of constraint of the arm against the chest, yielding a radial nerve palsy at the time of the temporary oligohydramnios caused by early amnion rupture. *F,* Unilateral leg hypoplasia with disruptive loss of postaxial rays in left foot (associated with gestation in a myomatous uterus). Note raised bony protrusion over left anterior tibia (? intrauterine fracture). (*B, C,* and *D* from Graham, J. M., Jr., Miller, M. E., Stephan, M. J., and Smith, D. W.: Limb reduction anomalies and early in-utero limb compression. J. Pediatr. 96:1052, 1980. *E* courtesy of Dr. J. Alan MacFarlane, Fairbanks, Alaska.)

22. POSTNATAL DEFORMATION

PREMATURE INFANT. The liability toward deformation depends on the magnitude and duration of the forces applied and the pliability of the fetus or infant. The prematurely born infant is more malleable than the term baby. In addition, the premature infant is more hypotonic and more likely to lie in one position persistently. If the surface on which he or she is lying is relatively firm, the premature infant will often develop flattening on both sides of the head, with a scaphocephalic, narrow head shape (Fig. 2–42*A* and *B*). In similar fashion, the thoracic cage may become relatively narrow in the anterior-posterior diameter. The risk for such deformations can be minimized to some extent by positioning premature infants on water-filled cushions, or "preemie waterbeds," instead of the usual relatively firm surfaces in standard incubators.

The premature baby may persistently lie on one side of the head and can develop a significant oblique-shaped (plagiocephalic) head as a result. This is particularly likely to occur in premature infants who undergo surgical procedures that limit the opportunities for repositioning or in neurologically-damaged infants. Obviously, gentle physical therapy and repositioning can help to prevent such postnatal deformations in premature infants.

FULL-TERM INFANT. A term infant with a neurologic deficiency or one who is seriously neglected may tend to lie in one position and may develop asymmetric flattening on one side of the head.

Torticollis may develop postnatally, especially when there has been injury to the sternocleidomastoid muscle at birth. Such infants may develop plagiocephaly and require helmet therapy for correction.

Thumb sucking seldom causes deformation in early infancy. However, once the teeth have developed, thumb sucking can deform the upper jaw. This is especially true when the child "pulls out" on the teeth.

Growth of the mandible tends to catch up to that of the maxilla during the first few years, and the mandibular teeth normally conform to the maxillary teeth. Supernumerary teeth or absence of teeth can lead to mild deformation, including malocclusions between the maxilla and mandible. Nowhere have the principles of mechanical treatment been more effectively employed than in the mouth. Once the teeth have fully erupted, they may be utilized as anchors for a variety of devices to alter the growth and/or alignment of the maxilla and/or mandible. Intraoral devices that provide rather small pressures on developing teeth can have a considerable impact on form.

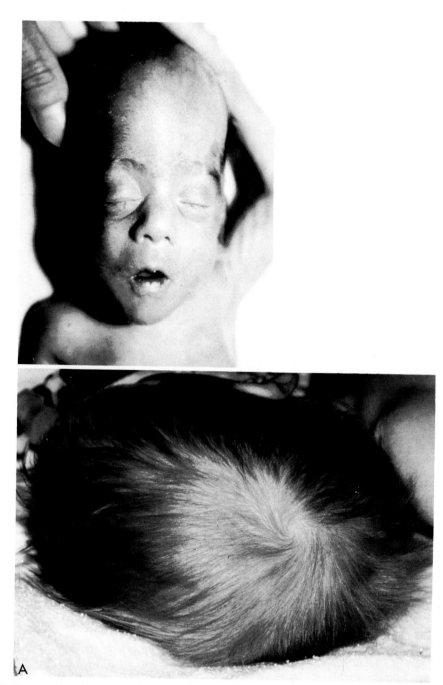

Figure 2–42. Postnatal deformation. *A*, Prematurely born infants with flattening of the head due to lying on relatively firm surfaces on one side of the head and then the other. Note that the impact is evident in the upper face as well.

Illustration continued on following page

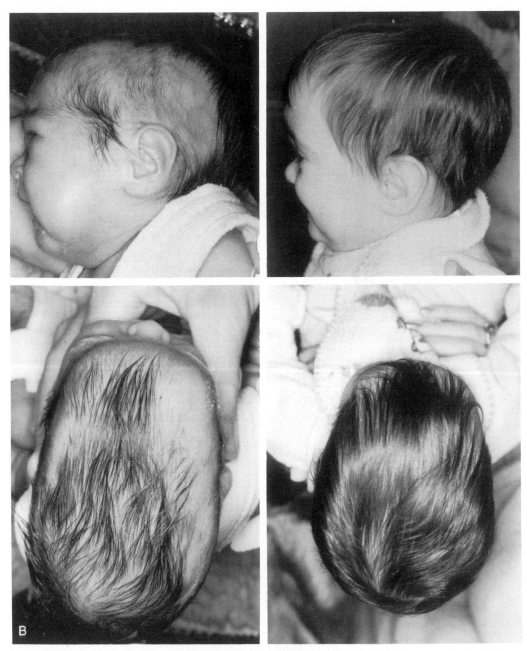

Figure 2–42 *Continued. B,* This infant was born at 31 weeks' gestation to a primigravida woman. This child was one of twins, born with oligohydramnios in vertex presentation, while her co-twin was in breech presentation with a normal amount of amniotic fluid. This twin had severe respiratory distress, while her co-twin had only mild respiratory distress. Marked dolichocephaly was evident at age six weeks (left), but this had resolved by age nine months (right).

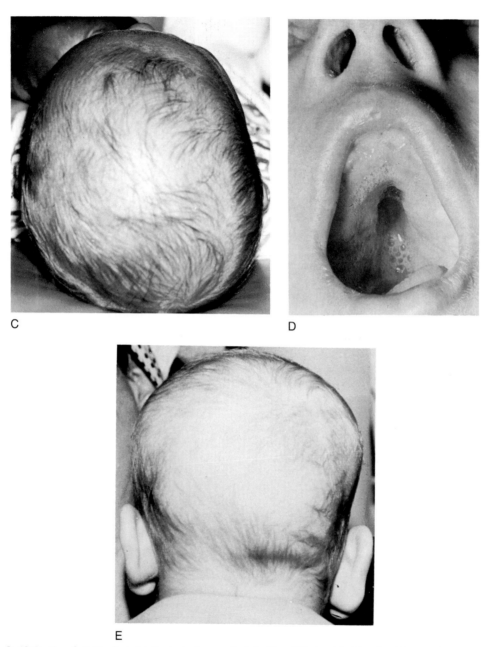

C

D

E

Figure 2–42 *Continued. C,* Neglected infant who lay on the left side of his head in his crib with secondary deformation toward an oblique shaped head. *D,* Middle-aged boy who is severely neurologically handicapped with a poor suck and swallow because of near-drowning at two years. Note the postnatal development of prominent lateral palatine ridges and a narrow palate, secondary to disuse. *E,* Impact of physical forces on the growth of auricle. This infant preferred to lie on the right side, and as a consequence the right ear was 0.5 cm longer than the left ear. (*D* and *E* courtesy of Kenneth Lyons Jones, M.D., University of California at San Diego.)

3

Clinical Approach to Deformation Problems

Mechanical forces are integral to morphogenesis, and unusual mechanical forces tend to yield unusual forms in developing tissues. The consequences are termed a deformation or deformation sequence.* The latter term refers to the manifold consequences of a single deforming cause, such as the oligohydramnios sequence. These types of defects are to be distinguished from malformations, in which there has been an intrinsic problem in the development of one or more tissues, and from disruptions, in which there has been a breakdown of a previously normal tissue.* This general classification of structural defects is summarized in Figure 3–1.

Given a structural defect that is presumed to be caused by aberrant mechanical forces, it is prudent to strive to determine whether the unusual forces were of extrinsic origin, affecting an otherwise normal fetus, or of intrinsic origin, resulting from a fetal problem such as a malformation. These two predominant modes of causation for deformation are shown in Figure 3–2. The distinction is based on a number of historical and physical findings. The major emphasis of this text is on extrinsic deformations due to in-utero constraint. Hence this category will be considered first, to be followed by the interaction of both extrinsic and intrinsic factors in the genesis of some deformations, and finally the intrinsic deformations due to a fetal malformation (Fig. 3–3).

EXTRINSIC DEFORMATIONS DUE TO UTERINE CONSTRAINT

The presumption in this category is that there is no primary problem within the fetus, but that the deformations are secondary to extrinsic forces that have deformed an otherwise normal fetus. The most common cause of extrinsic deformation is *uterine constraint*. About 2 per cent of babies are born with an extrinsic deformation; hence these are relatively common problems.[1, 2]

There is usually an adequate amount of amniotic fluid to cushion the fetus and allow

---

*The term sequence implicates the initiating defect plus its chain of consequences. For a malformation it implicates the initiating localized structural defect and any of its secondary consequences, some of which can be deformational. For a deformation it implicates the initiating *mechanical* aberration plus all of its secondary consequences. The word sequence was deemed more appropriate to convey this concept than the words syndrome (of which it may be a component), anomalad, or complex (synonymously utilized words in the past). Sequence was recommended for this usage by an international meeting on nomenclature organized by Professor Jürgen Spranger at the University of Mainz on November 10–12, 1979.

122

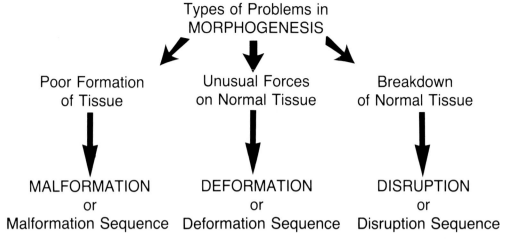

Types of Problems in
MORPHOGENESIS

Poor Formation
of Tissue

Unusual Forces
on Normal Tissue

Breakdown
of Normal Tissue

MALFORMATION
or
Malformation Sequence

DEFORMATION
or
Deformation Sequence

DISRUPTION
or
Disruption Sequence

Figure 3–1. The three predominant types of problems in the developmental pathology of structural defects.

full growth and mobility prior to 36 to 37 weeks of gestation (from conception). Thus, as Harrison and Malpas[3] indicated, one of the functions of the amniotic fluid is to distend the uterus and enable the fetus to move freely, to develop, and to grow with equal pressure in all regions with no excessive or localized constraint. As the fetus becomes crowded in its uterine "sac" during late gestation it will usually settle into a position in which the largest mobile fetal parts, the relatively bulky legs, have ample room. Thus the fetus tends to assume the vertex presentation. The implication that many of the extrinsic deformations are produced during late fetal life is supported by the observations of Nishimura,[4] who found that both dislocation of the hip and clubfoot are rare features in abortuses prior to 20 weeks of gestation.

After about 35 to 38 weeks of gestation, the human fetus tends to grow out of proportion to the uterine cavity, as is evident in viewing Figure 3–4. During this time the fetus is growing rapidly while the relative proportion of amniotic fluid is decreasing. The fetus thus becomes increasingly constrained. Uterine constraint of the rapidly growing malleable fetal tissues may result in mechanically induced deformations.

Since the cause of one deformation may often have led to other problems of constraint in the pliable fetus, there is a non-random occurrence of more than one deformation in the same child.[2] Dunn found that 30 per cent of newborn infants with a deformation problem had more than a single deformation. This non-random association of multiple deformations is summarized in Figure 3–5. A number of deformations consequent to the same extrinsic cause are referred to in this text as deformation sequences.

Uterine constraint tends also to reduce the rate of fetal growth and is one cause of prenatal growth deficiency. Such newborn

Figure 3–2. Unusual mechanical forces resulting in deformation may be the consequence of extrinsic constraint of a normal fetus or they may be the result of an intrinsic malformation of the fetus.

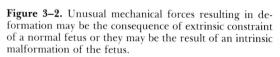

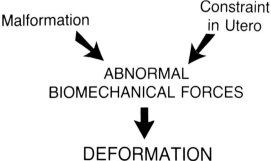

Malformation

Constraint
in Utero

ABNORMAL
BIOMECHANICAL FORCES

DEFORMATION

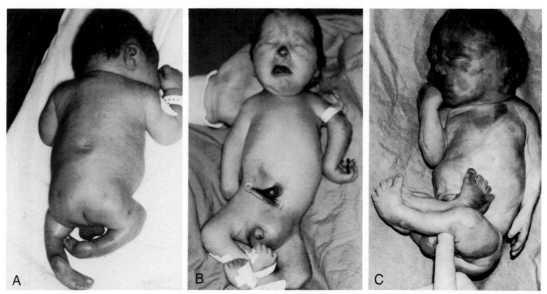

Figure 3–3. Intrinsic deformations due to congenital neuromuscular insufficiency are demonstrated in an infant *(A)* with sacral agenesis born to a mother with poorly controlled insulin-dependent diabetes, and an infant *(B)* with the amyoplasia form of arthrogryposis. Extrinsic deformations are demonstrated by an infant with oligohydramnios due to persistent leakage of amniotic fluid for the 6 weeks preceding delivery *(C)*.

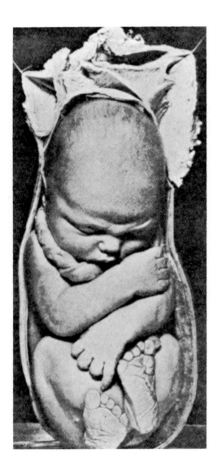

Figure 3–4. Term fetus of a primigravida in position to be born illustrating the uterine constraint that is a frequent feature in late fetal life. (The mother was killed in an auto accident and the fetus was dead on arrival at the hospital.) (From Peter Dunn, M.D., Southmead Hospital, Bristol, England.)

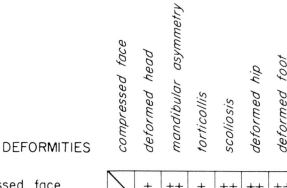

Figure 3–5. The non-random clinical association between deformations. (Adapted from Dunn, P. M.: Proc. R. Soc. Med. 65:735, 1972.)

DEFORMITIES

	compressed face	deformed head	mandibular asymmetry	torticollis	scoliosis	deformed hip	deformed foot
compressed face		+	++	+	++	++	++
deformed head	+		++	++	++	++	−
mandibular asymmetry	++	++		++	−	++	++
torticollis	+	++	++		++	−	++
scoliosis	++	++	−	++		++	+
deformed hips	++	++	++	−	++		++
deformed foot	++	−	++	++	+	++	

−not signif; + =p<0.05; ++ =p<0.001

babies frequently show deformational evidence of uterine constraint other than growth deficiency alone.

Any situation that tends to overdistend the uterus may be associated with early onset of labor and prematurity. This is a major concern for twins who simply distend the uterus prematurely and for the woman with a bicornuate uterus of the type that tends to become overdistended before term.

If the diagnosis is not clear at the time of birth the early postnatal course may provide valuable clues as to whether the deformations noted at birth are extrinsic in causation. The otherwise normal infant who has been constrained in late fetal life tends to show progressive improvement in growth and form after being released from the deforming situation at birth. If growth has been slowed by constraint in late fetal life, the infant tends to show catch-up growth toward his or her genetic potential in early infancy, usually within the first two months. If growth of particular parts has been restrained, they tend to show catch-up growth toward normal form. This was dramatically shown to be true

of nasal growth in an example of prolonged face presentation. Joints that have been externally constrained tend to show progressive increase in their range of mobility after birth.

If there is a lack of catch-up growth and/or return toward normal form after birth, then a further evaluation may be indicated to search for a more intrinsic problem within the patient that might be responsible for the deformation(s).

HISTORICAL PERSPECTIVE

During recent times there has been less recognition of mechanical constraint factors as a cause for problems of prenatal morphogenesis than was true during some periods in past history. As far back as Hippocrates it was noted that uterine constraint could cause fetal deformation.[1] Aristotle carried out experiments demonstrating that crowding of chick development caused limb deformation.[5] However, there was little written about constraint deformations from then until the Renaissance era. In 1573, Ambroise Paré of

France wrote that "narrowness of the uterus produces monsters by the same manner that the Dame of Paris carried the little dogs in a small basket to the end that they didn't grow." A little over a half century ago the text of *Diseases of the Newborn* by von Reuss[6] contained an entire chapter on postural deformations, whereas modern texts about the newborn have scanty coverage of this subject. One reason for the limited recognition of the more common mechanical factors in morphogenesis during the recent era may be the relative preoccupation with biochemical, molecular, and physiologic factors in morphogenesis. Though the latter are of obvious importance, so are the mechanical factors. This understanding is certainly important for the clinician dealing with problems of morphogenesis.

A number of investigators have made major contributions to our knowledge and understanding of extrinsic deformation during this century. A few brief summations and quotations from representative individuals will serve to emphasize some of their important observations and interpretations.

Thompson:[7] "We are ruled by gravity." "There is freedom of movement in the plane perpendicular to gravitational force." "Gravity affects stature and leads to sagging of tissues and drooping of the mouth."

von Reuss:[6] This early Viennese neonatologist made the following statement about contractural deformities: " . . . the deformities occur probably most frequently from pressure on the part by the uterine wall; sometimes marks of pressure may be observed on the skin."

Chapple and Davidson:[8] Chapple and Davidson noted that the "position of comfort" of the deformed infant soon after birth tends to be that which had existed in utero. Repositioning the baby into the "position of comfort" may allow the clinician to more readily deduce the causative compressive factors that resulted in the deformation.

Browne:[9-11] Denis Browne, who was an orthopedist at Great Ormond Street Children's Hospital in London, recognized that deformed infants were often the product of an "uncomfortable" pregnancy, implying uterine constraint. He emphasized the need for controlled forces, utilizing functional growth, in the correction of such deformations.

Dunn:[1, 2] Peter Dunn, a pediatrician and neonatologist in Bristol, England, who has been responsible for the resurrection and extension of knowledge about extrinsic deformation, states that "intra-uterine forces capable of moulding the fetus increase throughout pregnancy as the infant grows, the mother's uterus and abdominal wall are stretched, and the volume of amniotic fluid diminishes. At the same time the ability of the infant to resist deformation also increases as the rate of fetal growth slows, the skeleton ossifies, and leg movements become more powerful. All these factors are, of course, themselves directly or indirectly under the influence of heredity and are involved in a dynamic interplay throughout fetal life. Nature plays her hand to the limit. The price paid for a larger and more mature infant at birth, better able to withstand the stresses of extrauterine life, is a 2 per cent incidence of deformities."

FACTORS THAT ENHANCE FETAL CONSTRAINT IN UTERO

Table 3–1 summarizes some of the factors that increase the likelihood of fetal constraint in utero, and these are presented in more detail below.

Primigravida

The first fetus may experience more constraint than later offspring because he or she is the first to distend the uterus and the mother's abdominal wall. As a consequence, most constraint types of deformations are more common in infants of primigravidas

Table 3–1. FACTORS THAT INCREASE THE LIKELIHOOD OF FETAL CONSTRAINT IN UTERO

MATERNAL— —	Primigravida Small maternal size Small uterus Uterine malformation Uterine fibromata Small maternal pelvis
FETAL— — —	Early pelvic engagement of the fetal head Unusual fetal position Oligohydramnios Large fetus, rapid growth Multiple fetuses

than in infants of multigravidas. Figure 3–6 shows the form of the uterus and surrounding region in a primigravida and in a multigravida, emphasizing the differences in shape and size of the tissues around the fetus. This greater magnitude of late fetal constraint in the primigravida is considered a major reason why the first born is normally smaller at birth than later born offspring. Though the first born tends to be 200 to 300 gm smaller than later offspring at birth, they are of comparable size by one year of age.[12] Thus the mild late fetal growth deficiency in the offspring of a primigravida is transient,

and they tend to rapidly "catch up" to their genetic pace of growth postnatally. Usually this catch-up is achieved within the first few months after birth. The first born is also more likely to become constrained in an unusual position, such as the breech presentation, and to have consequent deformations relating to such a position.

Small Mother

The smaller the mother in relation to fetal size, the greater is the liability of deforming

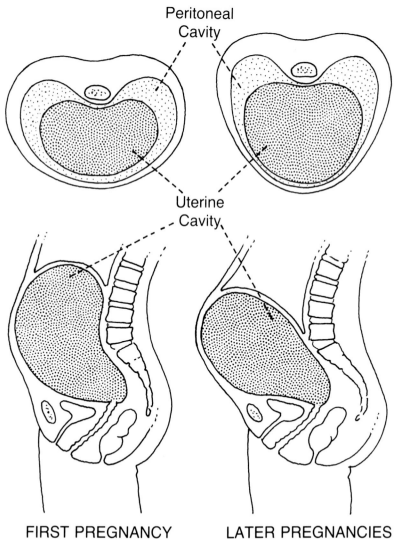

Peritoneal Cavity

Uterine Cavity

FIRST PREGNANCY   LATER PREGNANCIES

Figure 3–6. Diagrammatic transverse and sagittal sections of primigravida and multigravida abdomens to illustrate the impact of the unstretched abdominal muscles on the shape of the uterine cavity during the later weeks of pregnancy. (Adapted from Dunn, P. M.: Maternal and fetal aetiological factors. 5th European Congress of Perinatal Medicine, Uppsala, Sweden, 9–12 June, 1976, and Dunn, P. M.: Perinatal observations on the etiology of congenital dislocation of the hip. Clin. Orthop. *119*:11, 1976.)

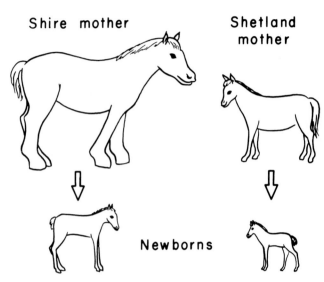

Shire mother

Shetland mother

Newborns

Figure 3–7. Influence of maternal size on the size of the offspring at birth is dramatically illustrated by the cross between a shire horse and a Shetland pony. Though the genetic situation is the same, the foal of the small mother is much smaller than that of the large mother, presumably because of the smaller space within which to rear the fetus. (Adapted from Hammond, J.: Growth in size and body proportions in farm animals. In Zarrow, M. X.: Growth in Living Systems. New York, Basic Books Inc. 1961, p. 321.)

uterine constraint in late fetal life. Thus most deformations are more common for the small woman than for the larger woman. The impact is readily evident in terms of birth size. Maternal size has a much greater impact on birth size than does paternal size. However, by one year of age the length of the infant relates equally to maternal and paternal stature.[12] Much of this maternal impact on birth size appears to relate to the transient effect of the smaller mother in restraining late fetal growth via uterine constraint. Postnatally the infant moves into his or her own genetic pace of growth, which is usually evident by one year of age. The effect of maternal size on prenatal growth is illustrated in Figures 3–7 and 3–8.

Uterine Malformation

Limitation in the capacity of the uterus to accommodate a fetus may result in early miscarriage, stillbirth, prematurity, and/or an offspring who survives to be born with sufficient constraint to give rise to deformation(s). Such reproductive problems are particularly likely to occur with uterine malformations such as a bicornuate or unicornuate uterus.[13] It is estimated that about 1 to 2 per cent of women have a uterine malformation. The likelihood of a deformation problem in the fetus reared in a bicornuate uterus has been crudely estimated to be about 30 per cent.[13] The recognition that a malformation of the uterus has caused a fetal problem may

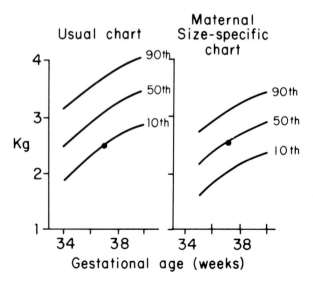

Figure 3–8. The weight of a 2.3 kg newborn baby born to a small mother with a weight of 40 kg and height of 150 cm, plotted on a usual grid (left) and on one that is specific for maternal size (right). (Adapted from Winick, M.: Biologic correlations. Am. J. Dis. Child. *120*:416, 1970. Standards to the right are from Thomson, A. M., et al.: The assessment of fetal growth. J. Obstet. Gynec. Brit. Comm. *75*:903, 1968.)

lead to corrective surgery of the uterus, thus providing a better opportunity for the next fetus to grow without as much constraint.

Uterine Fibromata

A large fibroid of the uterus may limit intrauterine space and therefore have gestational impact similar to that of a bicornuate uterus. The possibility of surgical removal of the tumor, allowing for better fetal space, merits consideration in such cases. Fortunately most uterine fibromata develop either late in reproductive life or after reproduction and are an infrequent cause of fetal deformation. However, a small fibroma may grow rapidly during gestation under the influence of increased levels of estrogen.

Small Maternal Pelvis

Vaginal delivery through a small pelvic outlet in relationship to the size of the fetus may result in appreciable molding of the craniofacies. This is usually quite transient. However, if there has been prolonged engagement of the fetal head into a small pelvis the degree of molding can be severe, and there may be a slower resolution toward normal form postnatally.

Early Pelvic Engagement of the Fetal Head

Early descent of the fetal head into the maternal pelvis is often accompanied by maternal symptoms of pelvic pressure and discomfort that sometimes include pains radiating down the legs while walking. It is very unusual for the fetal head to descend more than six weeks before term, and it seldom does so more than one month prior to delivery. Early fetal head descent is more common in the primigravida. When the symptoms are severe, it may be difficult for the mother to walk during the later period of gestation. The fetal consequences are predominantly craniofacial deformation. One potential result is vertex craniotabes,[4] which is secondary to prolonged compression of the top of the calvarium, resulting in poorly mineralized, malleable bone in the region of compression. Another potential consequence is constraint of fetal head growth in one dimension, resulting in a lack of growth stretch across one or more of the sutures. If there is a lack of growth stretch across a given suture, then that suture is more liable to become ossified and result in craniosynostosis.[15]

Fetal Position

Prior to 36 to 37 weeks from conception, when the fetus usually has adequate room for movement in its aquatic environment, it is not unusual for the fetus to be in varying positions, including breech presentation. As the fetus becomes more crowded, he or she will tend to shift into the vertex presentation position, there being more room in the fundal portion of the uterus for the bulkier legs.

Unusual late fetal position in utero may result from a number of factors, as summarized in Figures 3–9 and 3–10. This may be the consequence of a primary fetal neuromuscular problem, which limits the ability of the fetus to move in utero, and/or of a malformation that alters the form or function of the fetus. The more common reason for aberrant fetal position is in-utero constraint that has limited the capacity of the fetus to move into the vertex presentation. Abnormal fetal position during late fetal life may result in unusual constraint forces on fetal morphogenesis. Examples, which are set forth in Chapter Two, include breech presentation,

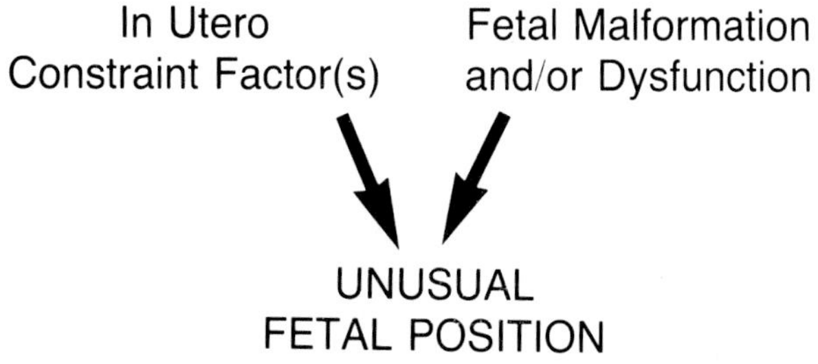

Figure 3–9. Unusual fetal position in utero may be the result of constraint factors to a normal fetus, or it may be the consequence of a primary fetal malformation and/or dysfunction.

In Utero
Constraint Factor(s)

Fetal Malformation
and/or Dysfunction

UNUSUAL
FETAL POSITION

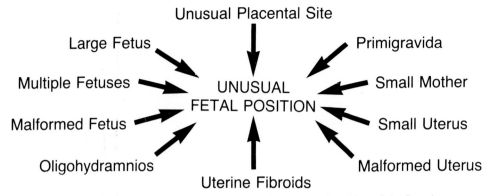

Figure 3–10. Maternal and fetal factors that can result in unusual position of the fetus in utero.

face presentation, brow presentation, and transverse lie. Breech presentation, though occurring only in about 4 per cent of pregnancies, is associated with about 32 per cent of all extrinsic deformations.[16]

Large Fetus, Rapid Growth

The fetus manifests a rapid rate of growth. For example, it doubles in weight during the six week period from 28 to 34 weeks in utero. The faster the growth rate and the larger the fetus, the greater is the liability toward external constraint types of deformation. The male is normally larger and grows more rapidly in late fetal life than does the female. Therefore, most extrinsic deformations are more common in the male than in the female, except for dislocation of the hip and other deformations that appear to relate to greater connective tissue laxity in females.

Multiple Fetuses

Multiple fetuses fill out the uterine cavity sooner than average. The average uterus is capable of handling about 4 kg of fetal mass. For twins this combined size is usually achieved by about the thirty-fourth week of gestation; thereafter there tends to be a slowing in growth as the uterine cavity becomes filled,[11] as shown in Figure 3–11. Other deformations besides transient growth deficiency also tend to be more common in twins, especially malpositioning of feet and molding of the craniofacies. This is one reason why monozygotic twins may not appear to be identical at the time of birth. One of the twins may have been constrained in a differ-

ent manner and to a different degree than the other twin. Some of this may relate to aberrant fetal positioning, especially the breech presentation in one of the twins.

Oligohydramnios

A deficit of amniotic fluid in late fetal life may be due to a variety of causes, such as early rupture of the amnion with chronic leakage of amniotic fluid, lack of urine flow into the amniotic space, or maternal hypertension. However, regardless of the cause, a lack of amniotic fluid tends to give rise to an unusual degree of uterine constraint, which affects fetal growth, including thoracic and lung growth, and may also cause a number

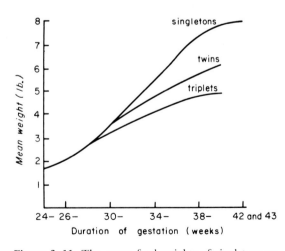

Figure 3–11. The mean fetal weights of singletons as compared to twins and triplets. While the initial growth rate is the same, the combined size of twins or triplets leads to earlier uterine constraint and late fetal slowing of growth. (Adapted from Bulmer, M. G.: The Biology of Twinning in Man. Oxford, Clarendon Press, 1970.)

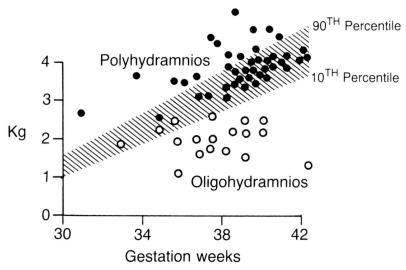

Figure 3–12. Impact on birth weight in kilograms of oligohydramnios due to renal insufficiency (open dots) versus polyhydramnios (solid dots). (Adapted from Dunn, P. M.: Growth retardation of infants with congenital postural deformities. Acta Med. Auxol. 7:63,1975.)

of craniofacial and limb deformations.[17] The consequences are referred to as the *oligohydramnios sequence*. The impact of oligohydramnios versus polyhydramnios on birth size is shown in Figure 3–12.

PROGNOSIS, MANAGEMENT, AND COUNSEL

When a deformation is due to external constraint in late fetal life in an otherwise normal individual, the prognosis for a return to normal form is usually excellent. The management of extrinsic deformations may vary with the cause. Sometimes it is worthwhile simply to observe the spontaneous changes for several days to several weeks after birth before making a decision as to whether any therapy is indicated. The mode of treatment may utilize corrective mechanical forces similar to those that gave rise to the deformation, in an effort to reshape the deformed tissues into a more normal form. When possible, this mechanical therapy should take advantage of normal growth. However, there should be caution in attempting to treat a deformation with a mode of management that may produce additional deformations.

The actual modes of management for reforming constraint deformations may vary appreciably and yet accomplish the same purpose. Simple manual manipulation with molding and stretching toward normal form

may be all that is needed. This is a common and ancient practice in India, where "massage women" are employed to mold and shape the baby. They come to the home daily for two to three months, or as long as indicated. By massage with oil and stretching, they form the baby into a normal shape and remove any extrinsic deformations that may have been present at birth. In a similar fashion, parents can be instructed to accomplish such molding or stretching at home. More consistent forces may be applied to foot deformities by frequent adhesive taping, with gradual improvement in the form. When such benign measures do not result in improvement, more rigorous means of molding and stretching, such as casting of the limbs or helmet molding of the head, may be utilized. When a joint is seriously dislocated or malpositioned and conservative measures have not been successful in accomplishing a repositioning to normal form, surgical intervention may be indicated. Ideally, this should be done as soon as it is established that conservative measures are not working. The tendency toward earlier surgery for such defects is especially important for congenital hip dislocation and for severe equinovarus deformity in which the calcaneus and talus are at least partially dislocated. Proper bony alignment is necessary to foster normal subsequent joint development.

The counsel given to parents of a baby with an extrinsic deformation problem can usually be quite favorable. With rare exceptions the parents may be counseled in the following manner: "I believe your baby is normal. He (or she) became crowded in the uterus before birth and this resulted in the somewhat unusual features at birth. Having been released from this constraint, the baby's features will return toward normal with no after effects. It is for this reason that I say your baby is normal." Any treatment that is merited is then explained to the parents, as is the recurrence risk. The recurrence risk depends on the cause of the extrinsic deformation. For most deformations, the recurrence risk is low. However, it may be quite high if the cause is a persisting one, such as a uterine malformation.

Obviously, it is important to distinguish between an extrinsic deformation and an intrinsic deformation problem secondary to a malformation, since this distinction has a major impact on the prognosis and management of the child and on the recurrence risk for the parents.

PREVENTION

At first thought, the prevention of extrinsic deformation seems an unlikely possibility. However, there already exist several examples of preventive measures, and more may be developed in the future. Surgical repair of a malformed uterus that has been shown to cause serious problems for fetal survival and deformation[13] may be followed by a greatly improved prognosis for a normal offspring.

A more controversial preventive measure is external version of the fetus who is in an aberrant position in utero. This is usually accomplished (by those rare physicians who practice external version) by 34 to 35 weeks from conception. After 35 weeks of gestation it is more difficult to accomplish external version of the fetus into the vertex presentation. The most common potential indication for external version is breech presentation. In the experience of one obstetrician who routinely practices external version for malposition in utero,[18] there has been a 0.54 per cent incidence of breech presentation at term. This is much less than the 3.5 per cent general frequency of breech presentation at term when external version has not been utilized. Since breech presentation has been considered responsible for almost one third of the extrinsic deformations and one half of the cases of dislocation of the hip in Dunn's series of some 6000 babies,[16] any reduction in the frequency of breech presentation at term might have quite an impact on the frequency of deformations, especially dislocation of the hip. However, there are risks involved in the procedure of external version, and it is a technique that is not routinely taught. Dr. Brooks Ranney of Yankton, South Dakota, has performed external version on about 10 per cent of 7000 pregnant women. He utilizes external version as early as the twenty-eighth week of gestation but more commonly at 30 to 34 weeks. Approximately 20 to 30 per cent of the fetuses revert, and external version is again carried out, up to as many as eight times. The contraindications to external version include multiple pregnancy, placenta previa, unicornuate uterus, and gross obesity. Anesthesia is never used. The version is accomplished by gentle maneuvering while monitoring the fetal heart. Dr. Ranney has not had any fatality related to the procedure. Hopefully, more studies will be done to determine whether the value of external version of the malpositioned fetus in utero is greater than any harm that may be done by the procedure. This question has not been fully resolved at this time, and the majority of obstetricians do not utilize external version in their clinical practices.

Prevention of the serious problems that are secondary to constraint deformation merits comment. One example is the scaphocephalic head with prominent occiput that may develop following prolonged breech presentation in late fetal life.[19] This so-called breech head is itself usually a benign deformation that tends to resolve postnatally. However, the contour of this head can pose serious problems during vaginal delivery because it tends to become arrested during the second stage of labor. This complication increases the liability for damage to the brachial plexus and cord trauma with neurologic residua during a vaginal delivery. Detection of the breech head by ultrasonography or radiography may warrant cesarean section delivery of such a fetus in breech presentation. Thus, prenatal detection of such a deformation may influence management toward prevention of serious vaginal birth trauma.

INTERACTIONS BETWEEN EXTRINSIC AND INTRINSIC FACTORS YIELDING DEFORMATION

A given deformation might relate to both extrinsic and intrinsic factors, representing an interaction between the two. One example is dislocation of the hip (Fig. 3–13). According to the author's judgment, most instances of dislocation of the hip are secondary to external constraint, which forces the head of the femur out of its socket and stretches the joint capsule and ligamentum teres. Dislocation of the hip is hypothesized to be more common in the female because the female fetus has more laxity of connective tissue than the male. This is presumed to be the consequence of a lack of testosterone in the female fetus, the assumption being that the testosterone yields tougher connective tissue in the male fetus.[20] Dislocation of the hip may also result from an intrinsic abnormality in the fetus having unduly lax connective tissue.[21] This can usually be discerned clinically by noting laxity in other joints in a patient with dislocation of the hip.

Another example of the interaction between intrinsic and extrinsic factors in creating a deformation is the fetus who has an intrinsic problem, such as a neuromuscular abnormality, that limits the ability of the fetus to turn into the vertex position before birth. Such a fetus is more likely to be caught in the breech position and to be born with such problems as breech head, dislocation of the hip, and other deformations that are more likely to occur in the fetus who is in the breech position.

INTRINSIC CAUSATION OF DEFORMATION

The cause of a given deformation may be altered mechanical forces as the consequence of a more *primary* problem within the fetus, such as a malformation. Although these intrinsic deformations are not the main subject of this book, it is important to be aware of them in the differential diagnosis of extrinsic deformations. Some of these deformations may be caused by either extrinsic factors or intrinsic ones. For example, the same type of malposition of the foot may be the consequence of external constraint of the foot, of neurologic deficit, or of a muscle disorder (see Fig. 3–3). The judgment of the clinician is required to determine the *primary* causation for the deformation. The overall diagnosis, prognosis, and recurrence risk counsel for the child with a malpositioned foot may differ widely if the deformation is secondary to uterine constraint rather than the result of a primary neuromuscular problem.

There are several types of intrinsic fetal problems that may result in altered mechanics and thereby give rise to deformation of otherwise normal tissues. Examples include neuromuscular disorders, aberrant growth of a tissue, and obstruction of a hollow viscus. Examples of each are set forth below.

Neuromuscular Problems

A deficit of neuromuscular function may result in multiple deformations. When the primary problem is neural, there may be a secondary loss of muscle mass. As a consequence of diminished movement, there may be joint fixations. Also, with a lack of stress the bone grows more slowly in breadth, tending to become more slender. This phenotype has been termed the fetal akinesia deformation sequence.[24, 25] Sites of muscle attachment to bone, which are normally prominent, may be less prominent or even lacking as a result of the neuromuscular deficiency.

Excessive neuromuscular function, such as

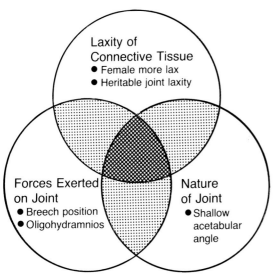

Figure 3–13. Interacting factors may relate to the liability to develop a deformation such as dislocation of the hip.

spasticity, may give rise to unusual magnitude and direction of muscle forces with consequent mechanical effects on morphogenesis.

Localized Growth Deficiency

Localized growth deficiency of one tissue may give rise to subsequent deformational problems in adjacent tissues. One such example is localized growth deficiency of the mandible. If this occurs in early morphogenesis it tends to place the tongue in a posterior location in the oropharynx. If this happens before nine to ten weeks of fetal life, prior to closure of the palatal shelves, the tongue may obstruct full palatal shelf closure, yielding a U-shaped palatal defect.[22] Once the baby is born there may be upper airway obstruction secondary to the retroplaced tongue. The combined findings are referred to as the Robin malformation sequence, previously called the Pierre Robin syndrome. Beyond the initiating malformation of a small mandible, the remaining features are deformations, the consequences of altered biomechanics engendered by the small mandible.

Localized Overgrowth

A localized overgrowth may cause mechanical problems in the adjacent region. This is obvious with most tumors. One example is a nasopharyngeal teratoma, which can obstruct palatine closure and partially occlude the upper airway, yielding deformational features similar to those noted for the Robin sequence.

Obstruction of a Hollow Viscus

Obstruction of a hollow organ will result in altered mechanics with increased pressures and deformations of the expanded tissue as well as distortion of tissues that surround the enlarging hollow structure. Examples include obstructive hydrocephalus, intestinal obstruction, and obstruction in the urogenital system. One dramatic illustration is the urethral obstruction sequence shown in Figure 3–14, which has been more commonly termed the prune belly syndrome.[23] Most commonly the primary malformation is an obstruction in the development of the penile urethra. This

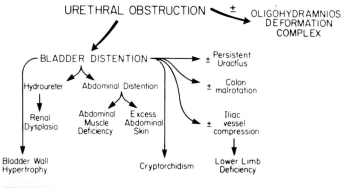

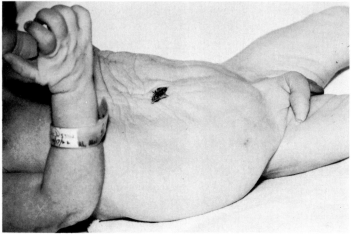

Figure 3–14. The development of the urethral obstruction sequence. The initiating malformation is most commonly urethral obstruction. All the other features are deformations due to the back pressure in the urinary system. In order to survive to a term birth the distended bladder must decompress, thus yielding the "prune belly" abdomen as shown below. (Top from Pagon, R. A., Smith, D. W., and Shepard, T.H.: Urethral obstruction malformation complex: A cause of abdominal muscle deficiency and the "prune belly." J. Pediatr. 96:900, 1979.)

results in massive enlargement of the bladder and the ureters. The back pressure adversely affects renal morphogenesis. The enlarging bladder distends the abdomen, causing diminished abdominal musculature. It also prevents full rotation of the gut, resulting in malrotation, and it obstructs full descent of the testes. The horrendous compressive effects of the distended bladder are usually lethal in early fetal life unless the bladder "blows out," either by rupturing an obstructing urethral valve or by way of the urachus, which tends to remain patent as a consequence of the pressure, or by rupture of the bladder or ureter. Once the bladder is decompressed, the fetus is left with a lax abdomen and redundant folds of excess skin, the so-called prune belly. Thus all these deformations are secondary to one primary intrinsic malformation, early urethral obstruction. Similar distention and muscular thinning of the abdomen can be seen with congenital ascites, which may result from a variety of causes.

The heart is a hollow viscus in which, as it develops, alterations in the direction or magnitude of blood flow, such as may be caused by partial obstructions, may give rise to secondary deformation in both form and size.[26]

References

1. Dunn, P. M.: The influence of the intrauterine environment in the causation of congenital postural deformities, with special reference to congenital dislocation of the hip. (Thesis for M.D. degree.) University of Cambridge, 1969.
2. Dunn, P. M.: Congenital postural deformities. Br. Med. Bull. *32*:71, 1976.
3. Harrison, R. G., and Malpas, P.: The volume of human amniotic fluid. J. Obstet. Gynaec. Br. Emp. *60*:632, 1953.
4. Nishimura, H., *In* Fraser, F. C., and McKusick, V. A. (eds.): Congenital Malformations. (International Congress Series, no. 204.) Amsterdam, Excerpta Medica, 1970, p. 275.
5. Tarruffi, C.: Storia della teratologia. (History of teratology.) Bologna, Regia Tipografia, 1881.
6. von Reuss, A. R.: The Diseases of the Newborn. New York, William Wood and Co., 1921.
7. Thompson, d'A. W.: On Growth and Form. A New Edition. Cambridge, The University Press, 1942.
8. Chapple, C. C., and Davidson, D. T.: A study of the relationship between fetal position and certain congenital deformities. J. Pediatr. *18*:483, 1941.
9. Browne, D.: Talipes equino-varus. Lancet *2*:969, 1934.
10. Browne, D.: Congenital deformities of mechanical origin. Proc. Roy. Soc. Med. *29*:1409, 1935–36.
11. Browne, D.: Congenital deformities of mechanical origin. Arch. Dis. Child. *30*:37, 1955.
12. Smith, D. W.: Growth and Its Disorders. W. B. Saunders Co., Philadelphia, 1975.
13. Miller, M. E., Dunn, P. M., and Smith, D. W.: Uterine malformation and fetal deformation. J. Pediatr. *94*:387, 1979.
14. Graham, J. M., and Smith, D. W.: Parietal craniotabes in the neonate: Its origin and relevance. J. Pediatr. *95*:114, 1979.
15. Graham, J. M., deSaxe, M., and Smith, D. W.: Sagittal craniostenosis: Fetal head constraint as one possible cause. J. Pediatr. *95*:747, 1979.
16. Dunn, P. M.: Breech presentation. Maternal and foetal aetiological factors. 5th European Congress of Perinatal Medicine, Uppsala, Sweden, 1976, p. 76.
17. Thomas, I. T., and Smith, D. W.: Oligohydramnios, cause of the nonrenal features of Potter's syndrome, including pulmonary hypoplasia. J. Pediatr. *84*:811, 1974.
18. Ranney, B.: The gentle art of external cephalic version. Am. J. Obstet. Gynecol. *116*:239, 1973.
19. Haberkern, C. M., Smith, D. W., and Jones, K. L.: The "breech head" and its relevance. Am. J. Dis. Child. *133*:154, 1979.
20. Arena, J. F. P., and Smith, D. W.: Sex liability to single structural defects. Am. J. Dis. Child. *132*:970, 1978.
21. Carter, C. O., and Wilkinson, J. A.: Joint and environmental factors in the etiology of dislocation of the hip. Clin. Orthop. Rel. Res. *33*:March–April, 1964.
22. Hanson, J. W., and Smith, D. W.: U-shaped palatal defect in the Robin anomalad: Developmental and clinical relevance. J. Pediatr. *87*:30, July 1975.
23. Pagon, R. A., Smith, D. W., and Shepard, T. H.: Urethral obstruction malformation complex: A cause of abdominal muscle deficiency and the "prune belly." J. Pediatr. *95*:900, 1979.
24. Moessinger, A. C.: Fetal akinesia deformation sequence: An animal model. Pediatrics *72*:857, 1983.
25. Hall, J. G.: Invited editorial comment: Analysis of Pena-Shokeir phenotype. Am. J. Med. Genet. *25*:99, 1986.
26. Clark, E. B.: Functional aspects of cardiac development. *In* Zak, R. (Ed.): Growth of the Heart in Health and Disease. New York, Raven Press, 1984, pp. 81–103.

4

Mechanics in Morphogenesis: Principles and Response of Particular Tissues

PRINCIPLES IN BIOMECHANICS

Rather simple principles apply for the role of mechanical factors in morphogenesis. These are that the direction and magnitude of forces affect the form of the developing individual, as illustrated in Figure 4–1. Some of the factors that affect the magnitude and direction of forces are summarized in Table 4–1. One major influence on the nature and alignment of forces is *growth*. Thus, the rate and shape of growth in a particular basic tissue will determine the magnitude and direction of the forces it exerts on adjacent tissues. The plasticity of a tissue is another factor that affects its liability to be altered by mechanical forces. The tissues of the fetus are pliable and easily molded. Another major influence is tension or compression related to muscle pull, gravity, or local constraint. The orientation within many tissues is determined by such forces. For example, collagen fibers, the basic threads and fibers of connective tissue, align in the direction of stress (Fig.

4–2). The strands are spun out by the fibroblast cells under genetic direction, but the alignment of the fibrils in the extracellular space appears to be predominantly determined by mechanical forces. If there is no consistent direction of mechanical forces, the collagen strands are haphazardly arranged. Given a sustained direction of forces they become organized and woven in relation to those forces.

The general precepts of mechanical engineering are relevant to man, as is the nomenclature (Table 4–2). In many tissues there is an integral interaction between growth and the forces of tension and compression. This is readily evident in the relationship between muscle usage and the size of muscle mass. The greater the forces, the larger the muscle mass tends to become. In turn, the stress of muscle tendon pull on a bone affects the growth and form of the bone. The greater the pull of a muscle on a bone, the greater is the size of the bony promontory at the site of the tension on the bone. For example, the

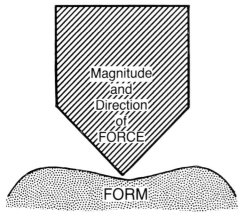

Depending on:
- Pliability of tissues
- Stage of development

Figure 4–1. The basic principles relative to deformation are simple—the magnitude and direction of forces have their impact on form. The response of a given tissue is dependent on its pliability and stage of development.

prominent bony ridge down the center of the skull in the male gorilla shown in Figure 4–3 relates to the size of the attachment of the powerful temporalis chewing muscles. The female gorilla does not have this prominent ridge because her muscles are less powerful.

We are ruled by gravity, which has a major impact on our form. Since our relative surface area to overall volume proportion is small, we are ruled by gravitational forces acting upon weight. In contrast, gravity is relatively negligible to very small animals that have a high surface area to volume ratio. Their world is more dominated by surface forces.

Examples of the impact of mechanical forces on morphogenesis abound in nature. The magnitude and direction of growth on form is dramatically reflected in the chambered nautilus, whose shell represents the successively larger living quarters occupied

Table 4–1. FACTORS AFFECTING THE MAGNITUDE AND DIRECTION OF MECHANICAL FORCES

External resistance to growth and/or movement
Growth rate and shape of basic tissues
Forces of fluid flow (or pressure)
Plasticity of fetus
Forces of muscle pull
Forces of gravity

by this mollusk as it outgrows and creates one new chamber after another, resulting in an equiangular logarithmic spiral shell, as shown in Figure 4–4. This also exemplifies the basic orderliness of the growth and its biomechanical consequences on the form of the organism.

Another beautiful example from nature of the impact of the size and direction of forces on form is the alignment of cellulose fibers in a tree. The reason the tree grows straight up relates to the cellulose fibers aligning in the direction of the stress force of gravity. Extrinsic forces, such as compression by snow during the winter, may deform the young tree. However, once released from such temporary constraint the sapling will again tend to grow in the direction of the force of gravity. The forces of prevailing winds may be sufficient to deform a tree. Controlled external forces may be utilized to deform a young tree into an aberrant form, a form that will be maintained after the tree is fully grown. Illustrative examples are shown in Figure 4–5.

The collagen fibrils within developing bone may be compared with the cellulose fibers of a tree. They are the basic structural elements and they align in the direction of stress in such a manner as to avoid shear forces, as previously indicated. This is dramatically evidenced in the longitudinal section of the human femur shown in Figure 4–6. The bone spicules are aligned in the direction of the stress of gravitational weight bearing and also of muscle pull. The form of the upper femur relates to the combined forces of weight bearing *plus* the pull of major muscle groups. This results in a sloping "neck" of the femur and the two large promontories of bone, the greater and lesser trochanters, in this region of the femur. The force lines that are evident in the form of such a bone may be of value to the engineer in his or her design of somewhat similar structures. D'Arcy Thompson[1] relates the story of a Zürich engineer, Professor Culmann, who became famous for his design of a mechanical crane. In the design of his crane he utilized stress forces that he observed in a longitudinal section of the human femur in 1871. When shown the section of the femur by his friend, Professor Hermann von Meyer of the Anatomy Institute of the University of Zürich, Professor Culmann exclaimed, "There is my crane!" Possibly, there should be a

NO DIRECTIONAL FORCES

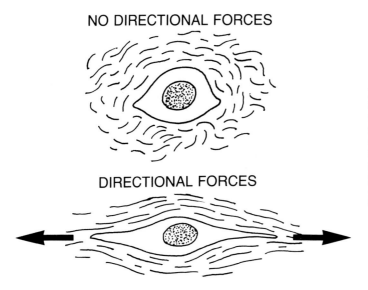

DIRECTIONAL FORCES

Figure 4–2. Schematic depiction of fibroblasts producing collagen fibrils. When there are no directional forces the extruded fibrils tend to be haphazardly oriented (above). When there are directional forces, the collagen fibrils align in the direction of the forces, thus affecting the form of the tissue. (From discussions with Prof. Gian Töndury, Anatomisches Institute, University of Zürich.)

closer interchange between biology and engineering, since the biomechanically determined "lines of stress" are naturally evident in many living creatures. The differences in these lines of stress will vary with the function of a bone. In the wings of a soaring bird, such as the vulture, the lines of stress relate to forces above and beneath the wing. The bone form in the pneumatized bone of the vulture is aligned accordingly and appears remarkably similar to the form that engineers learned to utilize in the wing girders of early airplanes and in bridge trusses, as shown in Figure 4–7.

Mechanical forces play a major role in the form of an individual and relate to the function of the individual. An example is the pneumatized lightweight but strong bones of the larger soaring birds. The largest soaring mammal, the extinct pteradon shown in Figure 4–8, had a wing span of 7 meters. It apparently had pneumatized wing bones. The form and dimension of the reconstructed pteradon are considered aerodynamically ideal for the soaring function of

this animal. Because its femora were delicately built and could not withstand compressive stress, it was necessary for it to hang upside down from cliffs as compensation for reduction in weight for flight. This adaptation is also true of the bat.

The evolutionary impact of forces upon form is also beautifully evidenced in the form of three different classes of creatures who came to live in the sea, as shown in Figure 4–9.

Abnormal mechanical forces give rise to deformation in man in much the same fashion as abnormal forces may deform a tree. In addition to those extrinsic deformations that relate to uterine constraint, abnormal forces can be seen in the deformations wrought by past societies in the name of beauty or custom by application of external forces after the time of birth, as shown in Figure 4–10A. Constraint forces were utilized to mold the head by a number of groups, including the "Flathead Indians," whose name derived from the practice. In the past, the Chinese custom of binding the feet of infant girls resulted in small and misshapen feet (Fig. 4–10C). In some societies the insertion of stretching devices into the ear lobes resulted in excessive skin in this region, as did similar practices with the lip. These techniques were designed to cause deformations. Other practices, such as the swaddling or papoose-board immobilization of infants, may have inadvertently increased the likelihood of deformation or hip dislocation.

Many types of cranial deformation were practiced in pre-Columbian Peru (Fig. 4–10D

Table 4–2. **MECHANICAL ENGINEERING TERMS THAT ARE APPLICABLE TO MAN**

Deformation—altered form due to unusual forces
Stress—intensity of force (force per unit area)
Strain—sufficient force to cause deformation
Tension—stretching forces
Compression—compressive forces
Torsion—twisting forces
Shear forces—forces contrary to the main orientation of a material or tissue

Text continued on page 144

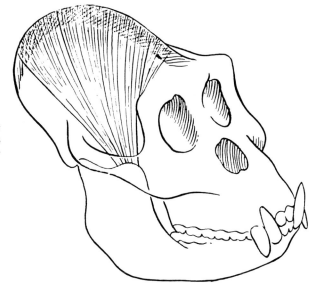

Figure 4–3. Male gorilla skull with prominent bony ridge down the center of the calvarium, which is the consequence of the pull of the powerful temporalis muscles, which insert at this location.

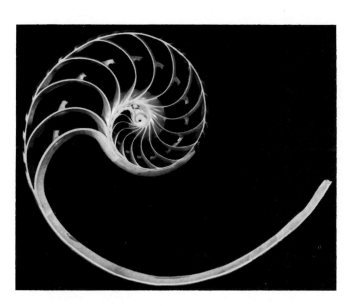

Figure 4–4. The growing nautilus mollusk outgrows one chamber after another, thus creating an equiangular logarithmic spiral shell.

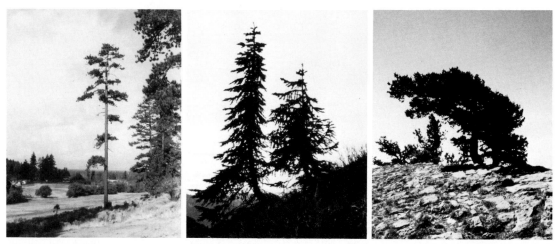

Figure 4–5. Left, Tree in a protected meadow location, growing stright up in relation to gravity. Middle, Alpine tree showing deformation of the lower trunk secondary to downward compression by the snow pack during the long winters in the early years of its growth. Right, Ridge-top tree showing deformation by the prevailing winds, which are from right to left.

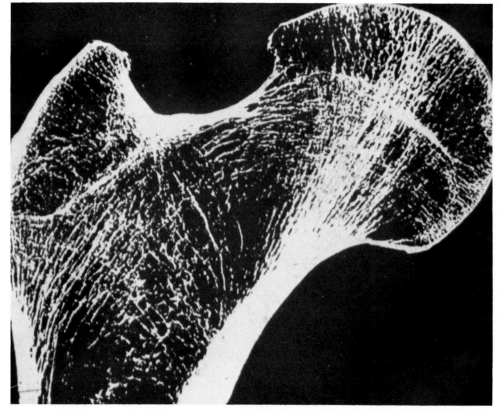

Figure 4–6. This section of the proximal human femur beautifully illustrates the relationship between function and form in the alignment of the bone spicules, which relate to the orientation of collagen fibrils. (From Thompson, d'Arcy: On Growth and Form. A New Edition. Cambridge, The University Press, 1942.)

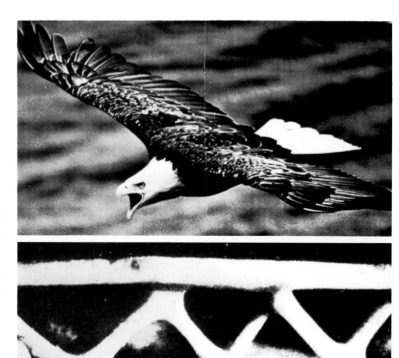

Figure 4–7. In the pneumatized bone in the wing of the soaring vulture, such as in the bald eagle (above), the orientation relates to the direction of air forces from below and above the wing. This generates a truss type of orientation highly similar to that utilized in the wing girders of early airplanes. (Bottom, from Thompson, d'Arcy: On Growth and Form. A New Edition. Cambridge, The University Press, 1942.)

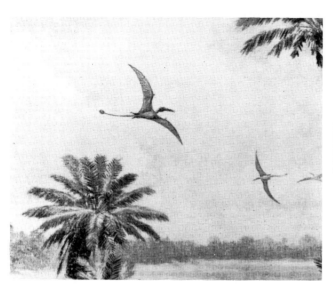

Figure 4–8. The form of the pteradon, related in ideal fashion to its function. (Courtesy of Ms. Pam Haas, American Museum of Natural History, New York City. Painting by Charles Wright.)

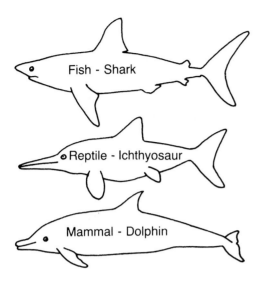

Figure 4–9. The adaptation of the form toward reducing turbulence and toward ease of free movement in water is beautifully exemplified by the similarities of form in a larger free swimming fish, a reptile, and a mammal. In this environment gravity is of less importance than is the buoyancy of the sea in shaping form. (Adapted from Bunnell, S., and McIntyre, J.: Mind in the Waters. New York, Charles Scribner & Sons, 1974.)

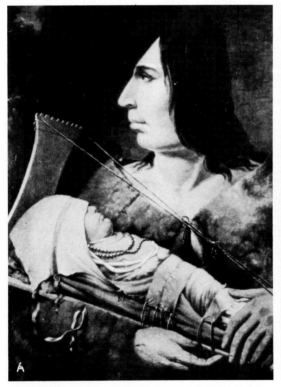

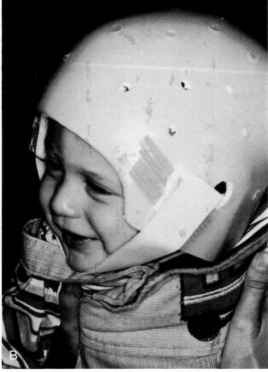

Figure 4–10. *A,* The Kwakiutl American Indians of the northwest utilized cedar boards and leather tongs to mold infants' heads. Boys were molded for five months, and girls were generally molded for seven months. (Courtesy of Bill Holm, the Burke Memorial Washington State Museum.) *B,* The same principles are used today to remold the heads of infants with plagiocephaly not associated with craniosynostosis.

Illustration continued on opposite page

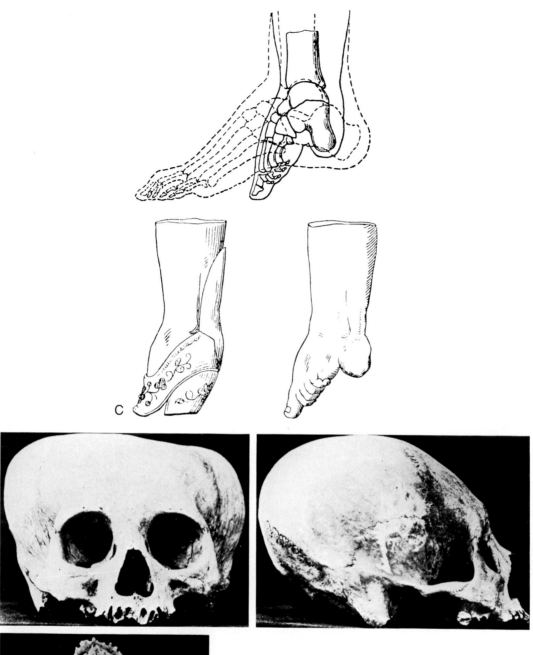

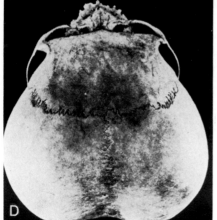

Figure 4–10 *Continued. C,* For almost 1500 years certain young Chinese girls were subjected to the harrowing experience of molding their feet several years in order to produce the desired small feet. These feet were deemed sexually attractive. The form into which the deformed feet were molded is shown above, and the special shoe and foot position is shown below. (From Levy, H. S.: Chinese Footbinding. New York, Walton Rawls, 1966.) *D,* This bilobed skull from highland Peru was created by application of a board to the occiput and a band over the sagittal suture and around the head.

Illustration continued on following page

143

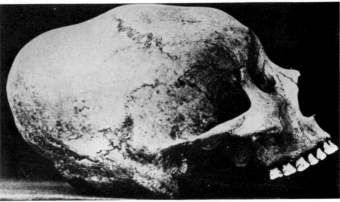

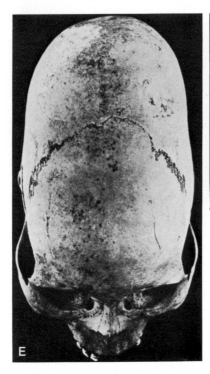

Figure 4–10 *Continued. E,* Highland Peruvians applied circumferential bandages to the calvarium.

to *F*).[2] Highland Peruvians applied circumferential bandages to elongate the calvarium. By combining banding with the application of occipital boards, skulls could be molded into a bilobed shape or a "tower-skull" configuration. Anthropologic observations suggest that the practice of artificial cranial deformation was quite widespread, occurring throughout the world.

Just as some past societies were knowledgeable about mechanical means of producing deformations after birth, so other societies successfully utilized biomechanical means to treat some congenital deformations. In India some women specialized in reshaping deformations by daily massage and manipulation. Among Polynesian societies, in which talipes equinovarus was a common deformity, there was usually an older woman who specialized in manipulating and binding such feet. The deformation was deliberately corrected only partially because such feet were ideal for climbing coconut trees and no shoes were needed in their environment!

MECHANICAL IMPACTS ON MORPHOGENESIS

Mechanical forces play an important role in the normal morphogenesis of most tissues.

Particular tissues have their own limited repertoire of responses to forces. The abnormalities mentioned in this section are utilized predominantly to illustrate more dramatically mechanical hypotheses that are relevant to normal morphogenesis of particular tissues. Many of the examples relate to the impact of forces during early morphogenesis, when extrinsic constraint deformation would be unlikely to occur. However, they do provide the reader with some clinically relevant illustrations of the impact of mechanical forces on form in morphogenesis.

Overall Growth

Constraint may limit the growth of the whole individual.[3] When the onset of constraint growth deficiency occurs during late fetal life there will usually be catch-up growth into the normal range once the constraint is relieved following birth. This appears to be the reason why the first born, who must distend the uterus and the mother's abdominal wall for the first time, averages about 200 to 300 gm smaller than subsequent offspring. The more the constraint, the greater is the deceleration of growth. This is dramatically evident in most multiple births. As shown in Figure 3–11, twins grow at a normal

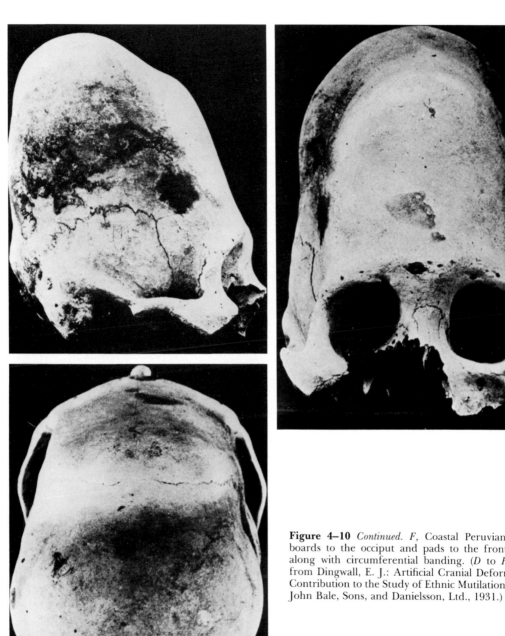

Figure 4–10 *Continued. F,* Coastal Peruvians applied boards to the occiput and pads to the frontal region along with circumferential banding. (*D* to *F* adapted from Dingwall, E. J.: Artificial Cranial Deformation: A Contribution to the Study of Ethnic Mutilation. London, John Bale, Sons, and Danielsson, Ltd., 1931.)

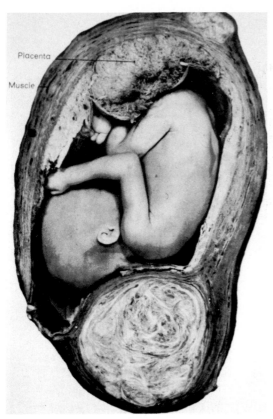

Placenta

Muscle

Figure 4–11. Diminished uterine cavity because of a large uterine fibroid.

rate for the first 30 to 34 weeks of gestation. After they have achieved a combined weight of 4.0 kg, they become constrained, and the growth rate tends to slow. The same types of phenomena have been noted in animal studies. If only one animal is reared in a uterine horn, the newborn is appreciably larger at birth than when many are reared in the same uterine horn.[4]

There are many other situations besides multiple births that limit the intrauterine space, causing it to yield a smaller baby. Examples include oligohydramnios, uterine malformation, and uterine fibroids. An example of the latter is shown in Figure 4–11.

Effects on Specific Tissues

Bone. The early cartilage models of the long bones appear to be genetically determined, but the alignment of collagen fibrils and of bone trabeculae relate to mechanical forces, as do the bony promontories. The alignment of collagen fibrils in the same direction as stress forces, thereby avoiding shear forces, has already been alluded to, as has the impact of the sites of muscle attachment on bone form. For example, the size and shape of the greater trochanter relates to the rather massive pull of five muscles at that site, including the very strong gluteus maximus muscle. The lesser trochanter has only one major muscle attaching at that site, the psoas minor. The combined forces of weight bearing plus muscle pull affect the form of the upper femur, including the normal "neck" of the femur. Prolonged muscle weakness in the growing child may give rise to less prominence of the trochanters and a straighter neck of the femur, a so-called coxa valga, as shown in Figure 4–12. It is important that these bony findings be interpreted as secondary deformations, the consequence of a more primary neuromuscular problem, rather than as additional malformations involving the skeletal system.

The impact of increasing weight is also evident on the breadth of bone. The strength of a leg bone, for example, depends on the area of its cross section. Since the legs must hold up a body that increases in weight by the cube of its height, they thicken much more in a heavy person than they do in a small person. Galileo first recognized this principle in his *Discorsi* in 1638. He reasoned that the bone of a large animal must thicken disproportionately to provide the same relative strength as the slender bone of a small animal.

Stress forces affect not only the form of bone but also the growth of bone. Linear growth is only mildly affected by muscle weakness. Thus, paralysis of a limb results in only a 5 to 10 per cent reduction in its rate of linear growth. However, subperiosteal growth in bone breadth is more dramatically affected. Hence, with muscle weakness or lack of use, the growing bone tends to become slender, as is shown in Figure 4–13.

The adaptive capacity of bone is beautifully exemplified by the realization that the amount of bone present and its alignment are influenced by the very forces that the bone is required to withstand. Bone appears to have a critical strain or stress threshold above which there tends to be bone deposition and below which there tends to be bone resorption. Intermittent stress on a bone tends to foster local growth of bone, as ex-

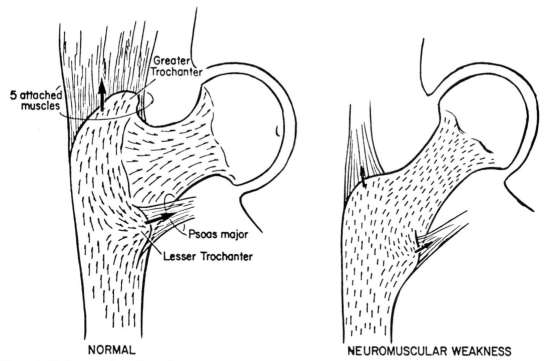

Figure 4–12. Impact of muscle weakness on the form of the proximal femur. The coxa valga and slimmer bone is secondary to the diminished forces exerted on the bone.

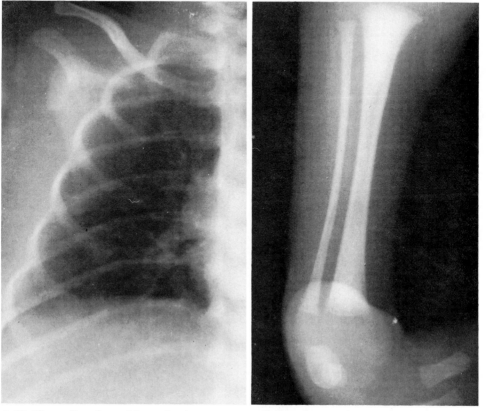

Figure 4–13. These slim ribs and lower leg bones are secondary to longstanding neuromuscular weakness in a newborn baby with myotonic dystrophy whose mother had this dominantly inheritable disorder.

emplified in bony promontories at sites of muscle attachment. One example is the bony spurs that are liable to develop in the arch of the foot as a result of the strain of long distance running. However, persistent stress on a bone, such as that caused by continuous external compression, can lead to a decrease in bone. This is dramatically exemplified by constraint vertex craniotabes. This abnormality appears most commonly to be secondary to prolonged constraint pressure on the fetal head as a consequence of the head being forcibly "engaged" for a long period of time prior to birth.

A similar but postnatal type of impact of persisting pressure on the calvarium was deduced by G. E. Smith[5] from his evaluation of ancient Egyptian skulls. He recognized that the upper class Egyptians who lived during the fourth to the nineteenth dynasties and wore heavy headdresses had a peculiar thinning of the calvarium. Smith deduced that this was the consequence of the *continuous pressure* exerted by these heavy headdresses.

Joints. Joints develop secondarily within the condensed mesenchyme of the developing bones. Movement is an important factor in joint morphogenesis. A chronic lack of movement tends to give rise to joint contracture.[6] One dramatic example was an infant with multiple joint contractures (termed arthrogryposis) whose mother had received tubocurarine for 19 days in early pregnancy for the treatment of tetanus.[7] The medically induced early immobilization for 19 days was considered to be the cause of the joint contractures in the fetus. Similar defects have been induced experimentally by Moesinger[8] by injection of curare into pregnant mice. The consequent defects have been termed the fetal akinesia sequence (Fig. 4–14). Physical constraint may also yield joint contractures. Figure 4–15 demonstrates the multiple consequences on bones and joints in markedly constrained twins carried to term by a small primigravida woman.

Muscles. Muscle cells align in the direction of muscle pull. In addition to avoiding shear forces, this has obvious importance to muscle function. The size of the muscle relates to the magnitude and frequency of the forces: the larger the forces, the greater is the muscle bulk. Conversely, with diminished function, the muscles become smaller in size. A lack of any function will result in a diminished, hypoplastic muscle. The biomechanical impact of muscle strength on bone form and growth has already been emphasized.

Organ Capsules. Organ capsules may be viewed as exoskeletons that provide connective tissue support for particular tissues. Included within this category are the dura mater of the brain, the sclera and outer covering of the eye, the pericardium of the heart, the pleura of the lung, the peritoneum of the intestine, the capsule of the kidney, and the tunica albuginea of the testes. The skin may also be interpreted as an organ capsule: it is the capsule for the entire organism. The only organ capsule that becomes ossified is that of the brain. The dura mater is responsible for the development and ossification of the calvarium; this will be considered in more depth in the craniofacial section. None of these organ capsules appear to have any basic impetus for growth. Rather, they grow in accordance with the mechanical forces imposed by the expansion of the particular organ or tissue that they envelop. All the organ capsules are composed of connective tissues within which the collagen fibrils align in accordance with the growth stretch imposed by the internal expansile growth of the respective organ. The direction of such forces is curvilinear, as is readily evident in the alignment of the collagen fibrils within these organ capsules.

Skin and Its Derivatives. Skin does not appear to have any basic impetus for growth, but grows in accordance with mechanical forces.[9] Normally the forces are exerted by the growth of underlying tissues. If there is unusual growth of underlying tissues, the skin will respond accordingly. Thus, if there is hydrocephalus, the skin will grow in accordance with the enlarged head. The excessive skin of the "web neck" that may occur in XO Turner syndrome and other disorders is considered secondary to a more primary problem in the development of the lymphatic system, as shown in Figure 4–16. A defect in communication between the jugular lymph sac and the internal jugular vein results in a grossly distended jugular lymph sac that increases the growth of the skin in that posterolateral region of the neck.[10] The lymphaticovenous communication usually develops before the time of birth, thus draining the distended lymphatic sacs. The excess skin remains as a redundant fold from the mastoid region toward the shoulder, a deformational clue to the nature of the problem that

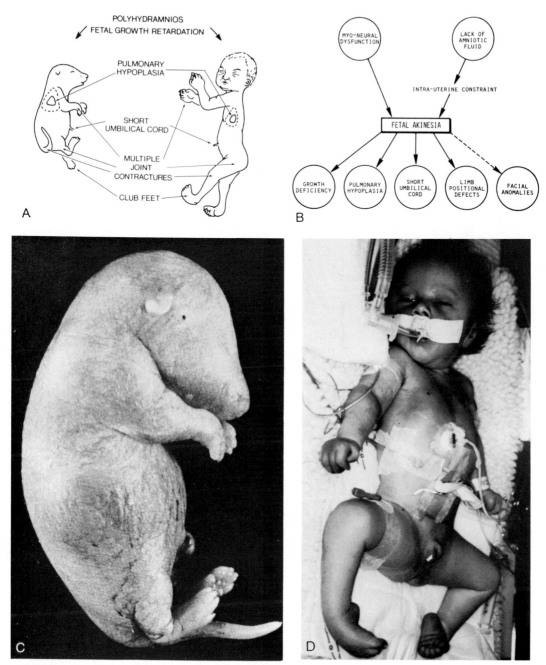

Figure 4–14. The fetal akinesia sequence *(A* and *B)* results from decreased in utero movement. This condition has been produced experimentally in fetal rats *(C)* that were curarized from day 18 of gestation until term (day 21). The consequent anomalies consisted of intrauterine growth retardation, micrognathia, multiple joint contractures, pulmonary hypoplasia, short umbilical cords, and polyhydramnios. These defects in the fetus can result from intrinsic deformation due to myoneural dysfunction (associated with smooth, tight skin and polyhydramnios due to lack of swallowing amniotic fluid) or extrinsic deformation due to oligohydramnios resulting from a number of causes (and usually associated with skin redundancy). The infant in *D* has the fetal akinesia deformation sequence due to Type I Pena-Shokeir syndrome, an autosomal recessive disorder that was lethal in this child and a subsequent sibling due to pulmonary hypoplasia. *(A, B,* and *C* from Moessinger, A. C.: Fetal akinesia deformation sequence: An animal model. Pediatrics 72:857, 1983.)

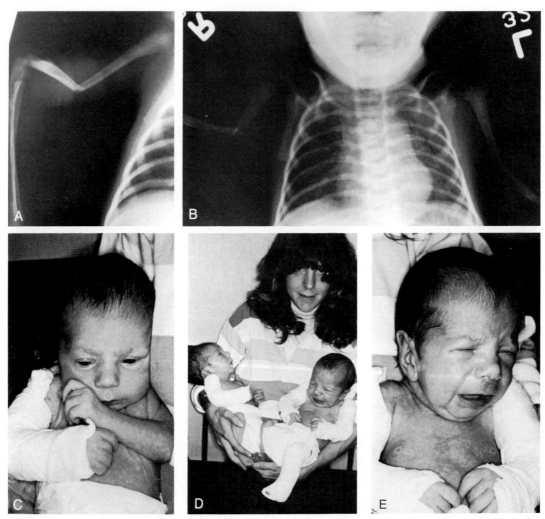

Figure 4–15. This 5 ft 2 in, 98-lb primiparous mother clearly had her hands full when these twins were born at term with a combined weight of 10 lb, 11 oz. There was marked fetal crowding during the last half of gestation to the extent that this small mother had difficulty eating because of "bloating," resulting in a 2-lb weight loss during the course of the pregnancy. The mother noted very little fetal movement during the third trimester, and both twins were born with severe joint contractures ("arthrogryposis"), resulting in 60 to 90 degrees limitation of extension at the elbows and about 30 degrees limitation of extension at the knees. Twin A (*A* and *C*) was born from a vertex presentation with thin bones, resulting in a fracture postnatally during routine handling. Twin B (*B* and *E*) was delivered vaginally from a breech presentation with thin bones and fractured both humeri during delivery; he also had a right equinovarus foot deformity. Both twins had markedly redundant skin and large ears as a consequence of prolonged compression. By the time photographs *C, D,* and *E* were taken (at 12 days old), the joint contractures had shown marked improvement, and the twins were beginning to fill out their loose skin. It is difficult to imagine how they fit into this petite mother (*D*). The prognosis for continued improvement is excellent.

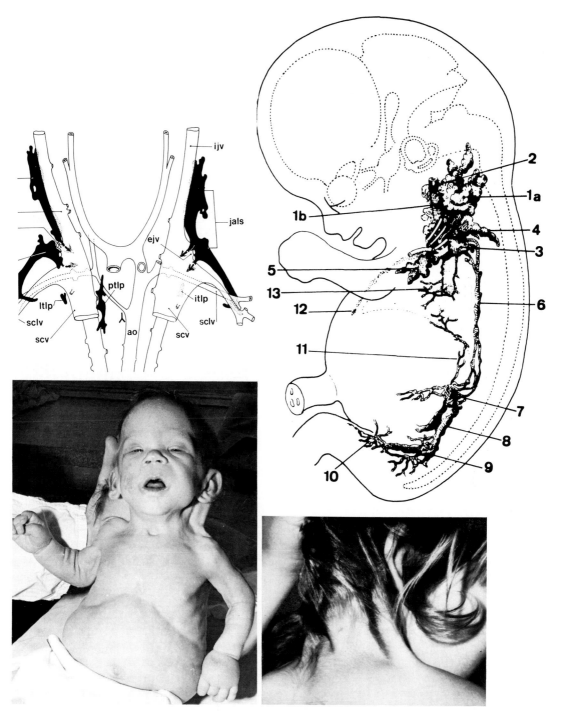

Figure 4–16. Upper right, The early developing lymph channels drain into the venous sytem. In the cervical region the jugular lymph sac (1a) drains into the jugular vein (2) at the site designated 1b. This is shown in the upper left at 40 days of development, by which time the communication (arrows) from the jugular and axillary lymph sacs (jals) has occurred into the jugular vein.

Upper left, If there is a delay or failure in the development of the communication between the lymphatic system and the venous system there is a damming up of the lymph, as was still evident at the time of birth in this XO Turner syndrome girl. The distended jugular lymph sac results in the growth of excess skin in the lateral neck. Once the lymph drainage has occurred, the individual is left with a residuum of redundant skin referred to as "web neck," shown at lower right in the same girl several years later. Lymph accumulation may yield peripheral lymphedema, and prior lymph accumulation may yield such residual features as loose skin in the face and a lax abdomen. (Upper right from Töndury, G., and Kubik, S.: Zur ontogenese des lymphatischen Systems. Handbuch der Allgemeinen Pathologie, Berlin, Springer-Verlag, 1975. Upper left from van der Putte, S. C.: The development of the lymphatic system in man. Adv. Anat. Embryol. *51*:1, 1975.)

engendered the web neck. Another condition that may leave a residuum of redundant skin is early urethral obstruction, which can massively distend the bladder in early fetal life.[11] This will usually be lethal early in fetal life unless the bladder decompresses, which will yield a wrinkled "prune belly" with redundant folds of abdominal skin at birth.

The skin appears to respond to external pressure by growth in a fashion similar to its response to internal expansile stretch. For example, when there has been external constraint on the skin, such as with oligohydramnios, there may be loose and redundant folds of skin at birth. Such accentuated folds in the face may account for the "Potter facies" noted with the external constraint due to oligohydramnios. Redundant loose folds have been noted on the back of the neck in infants who have been in prolonged breech presentation with the head hyperextended to yield the "breech head" deformation. This is presumed to be the consequence of excessive pressure of the basiocciput on the posterior neck resulting in localized overgrowth of the skin in this region. In similar fashion, skin overgrowth in an anterior neck and chin region may be noted with prolonged face presentation. Thus, the finding of redundant excessive skin at birth may implicate either past internal expansile growth stretch or past external compressive constraint of considerable duration.

An occasional finding in a normal baby is a small raw, punched-out lesion in the skin of the scalp. Such lesions also are a frequent feature in babies with the 13 trisomy syndrome, as shown in Figure 4–17, and occasionally in other disorders. They tend to occur in close proximity to the parietal hair whorl. The parietal hair whorl may represent the apical point from which growth stretch is exerted by the domelike outgrowth of the brain. This point in the developing skin of the scalp would therefore be the most liable to break down during the period of rapid brain growth, which stretches the skin away from this point. Under this hypothesis, the ulceration would be the result of the interaction of mechanical forces plus a greater than average liability to breakdown of the skin at this point of maximal stretch.[12]

1. Hair directional patterning: As the hair follicles grow down from the germinative layer of the skin at 10 to 18 weeks of development they come to have a sloping angula-

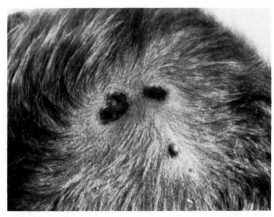

Figure 4–17. Small scalp ulcerations in a newborn infant with the 13 trisomy syndrome. Note that these lesions tend to occur at or near the site of the parietal hair whorl, the location of maximal stretch exerted on the developing skin of the scalp by the domelike outgrowth of the brain.

tion (Fig. 4–18).[13] This angulation is considered to be the consequence of the direction and magnitude of growth stretch exerted on the surface skin during the period of downgrowth of the hair follicles, which, as a result of differential lag, have a sloping angulation. When the keratinized rod of hair is finally extruded at 18 weeks of development, its hair direction appears to be set for life and reflects the magnitude and direction of growth stretch exerted on the skin during the 11 to 18 week fetal period (Figs. 4–19 and 4–20). On any expanding sphere or hemisphere there is one immobile point away from which all other points are moving. Over the scalp this is usually in the parietal region and is considered the genesis of the parietal hair whorl, or crown. This is a beautiful example of the impact of mechanical forces on form. Thus differences in brain growth and form are considered the reason for most differences in scalp hair directional patterning, including those that exist between humans and other primates, as shown in Figure 4–21. Of special clinical relevance are the aberrant hair directional patterns that may be secondary to problems of brain morphogenesis, examples of which are shown in Figures 4–22 through 4–25. Such findings not only tend to implicate a problem in brain morphogenesis but also suggest that the disorder had its advent prior to 16 weeks of fetal life.

2. Nails: Each nail is a keratinized plate which, as with hair follicles, is derived from

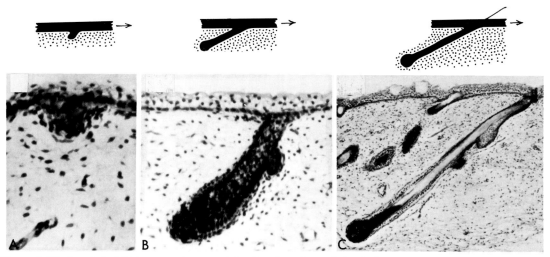

Figure 4–18. As a hair follicle grows downward, its direction of angulation is determined by the forces exerted via the underlying growth of the brain. These stretch forces, greater at the surface than in deeper tissues, affect the hair directional patterning, which is usually set by about 16 weeks. (From Smith, D. W., and Gong, B. T.: Scalp-hair patterning: Its origin and significance relative to early brain and upper facial development. Teratology 9:17, 1974.)

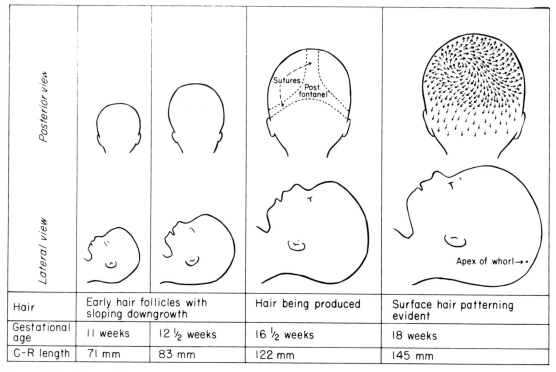

Hair	Early hair follicles with sloping downgrowth		Hair being produced	Surface hair patterning evident
Gestational age	11 weeks	12 ½ weeks	16 ½ weeks	18 weeks
C-R length	71 mm	83 mm	122 mm	145 mm

Figure 4–19. The rapid domelike projection of the brain during the period of hair follicle downgrowth is evident in these proportionate drawings of the early fetal head, during the era of hair follicle downgrowth. (From Smith, D. W., and Gong, B. T.: Scalp-hair patterning: Its origin and significance relative to early brain and upper facial development. Teratology 9:17, 1974.)

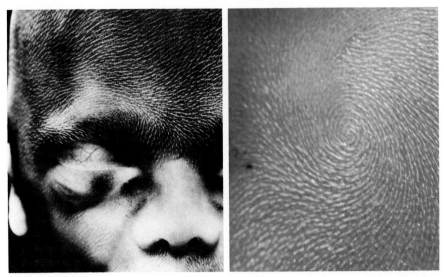

Figure 4–20. As the hairs emerge at about 18 weeks the hair directional patterns are beautifully evident. Left, Over the forehead the "frontal hair stream," emanating from the fixed skin points of the ocular puncta, meets with the downsweeping parietal hair stream, which emanates from the parietal whorl. Right, The parietal hair whorl (crown). On any expanding sphere or hemisphere there must be at least one fixed point from which all other points are moving. Presumably it is the mild asymmetry of forces that conveys the whorl pattern. (From Smith, D. W., and Gong, B. T.: Scalp-hair patterning: Its origin and significance relative to early brain and upper facial development. Teratology *9*:17, 1974.)

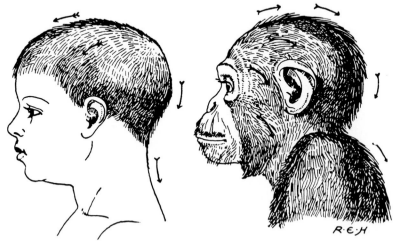

Figure 4–21. Head hair patterning in a boy versus that in a young chimpanzee. In the human, the large domelike brain has generated a parietal whorl and the hair "streams" from that spot, with the parietal hair stream sweeping forward to meet with the frontal hair stream on the forehead. Since the chimpanzee has a much smaller brain, the frontal hair stream simply sweeps directly back over the head with no parietal whorl or parietal hair stream. (From Kidd, W.: The Direction of Hair in Animals and Man. London, Adam and Charles Black, 1903.)

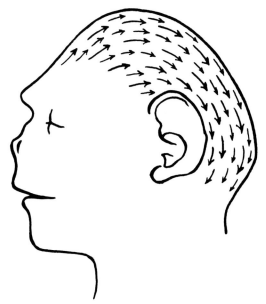

Figure 4–22. Child with severe microcephaly and midfacial defect. There is no parietal hair whorl and the frontal hair stream sweeps back over the scalp in similar fashion to that found in the chimpanzee (Figure 4–21). (From Smith, D. W., and Gong, B. T.: Scalp-hair patterning: Its origin and significance relative to early brain and upper facial development. Teratology 9:17, 1974.)

the germinative layer of skin. The nail tends to conform to the shape of the distal phalanx, as shown in Figure 4–26. Thus, if the distal phalanx is short and broad, the nail is short and broad. If the distal phalanx is narrow, the nail is narrow. If the distal phalanx is bifid, the nail is bifid. The impact of forces

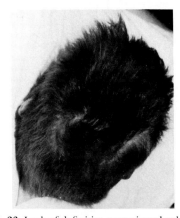

Figure 4–23. Lack of definitive posterior whorl in a child with severe microcephaly. (From Smith, D. W., and Gong, B. T.: Scalp-hair patterning: Its origin and significance relative to early brain and upper facial development. Teratology 9:17, 1974.)

on the early form of the nails is illustrated in Figure 4–27.

3. Dermal ridge patterning: As with other primates, man has dermal ridges on the thickened skin of the volar surface of the hand and foot. This parallel ridging provides an important frictional surface for the palm and sole. These ridges develop at 13 to 19 weeks of fetal life and appear to form at right angles to the plane of growth stretch in the skin.[14] Figure 4–28 illustrates the similarity to the ridges that develop in the sand of a beach at right angles to the direction of the flow of water or of wind. The surface characteristics where there are underlying pads give rise to curvilinear dermal ridge patterns that reflect the shape of the pads at the time of dermal ridge development (Figs. 4–29 and 4–30). If the fingertip pad is low, the patterning takes the form of an arch. However, if the pads are very prominent, a whorl is expected, with the center of the whorl representing the apex of the pad. A high proportion of loops, the more common fingertip patterning, is of little clinical relevance. The finding of six or more arches on the 10 fingertips is unusual (3 per cent of normal), and the finding of eight or more whorls on the fingertips is also unusual. Altered dermal ridge patterning is generally a nonspecific deformation, providing evidence of the nature of the topographical growth in the volar surfaces of the hands and feet at 13 to 19 fetal weeks.

4. Dermal creases: The dermal creases are simply deep wrinkles that reflect the flexional planes of functional folding in the thickened skin of the palms and soles,[15] as shown in Figure 4–31. They occur in relation to joints and provide evidence of the functional movement at such joints. Over the palm, the thenar flexional crease relates to the flexional plane of oppositional flexion of the thumb and first metacarpal. The upper palmar crease reflects the sloping plane of flexional folding of the third, fourth, and fifth metacarpophalangeal joints, and the mid-palmar crease simply reflects the folding plane in the skin between the other two palmar creases. By ever so small a difference in the shape or form of the hand it is possible to have a single upper palmar crease—the simian crease, as shown in Figure 4–32. This highly nonspecific finding is unilateral in 4 per cent of normals and bilateral in 1 per cent.

Craniofacial Region. The usual formation

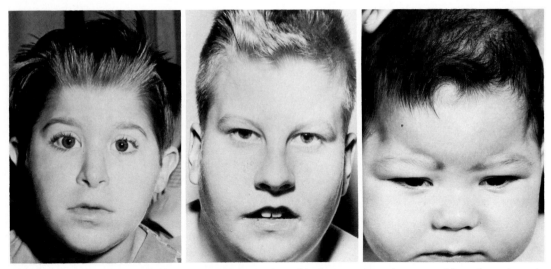

Figure 4–24. Frontal brain deficiency may result in the frontal hair stream sweeping upward into the scalp region and giving rise to a frontal upsweep, more commonly referred to as a "cowlick." Mild degrees of this occur in about 3 per cent of normal individuals. These represent unusual degrees in a child with Rubinstein-Taybi syndrome (left), Prader-Willi syndrome (middle), and fetal rubella syndrome (right). At the site of juncture of the upsweeping frontal hair stream and the downsweeping parietal hair stream there may be a convergent whorl, as shown to the right. (Left and middle from Smith, D. W., and Gong, B. T.: Scalp-hair patterning: Its origin and significance relative to early brain and upper facial development. Teratology 9:17, 1974. Right, courtesy of Dr. Patrick MacLeod, University of British Columbia.)

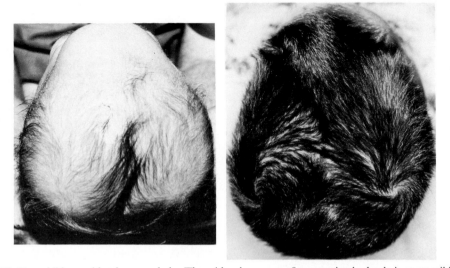

Figure 4–25. Two children with trigonocephaly. The wide placement of two parietal whorls is compatible with the developing brain having had an abnormal triangular shape prior to 16 weeks of fetal life. Five per cent of normal children have bilateral whorls, but they are spaced close to the midline in contrast to the situation in these two individuals. (From Smith, D. W., and Gong, B. T.: Scalp-hair patterning: Its origin and significance relative to early brain and upper facial development. Teratology 9:17, 1974.)

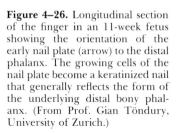

Figure 4–26. Longitudinal section of the finger in an 11-week fetus showing the orientation of the early nail plate (arrow) to the distal phalanx. The growing cells of the nail plate become a keratinized nail that generally reflects the form of the underlying distal bony phalanx. (From Prof. Gian Töndury, University of Zurich.)

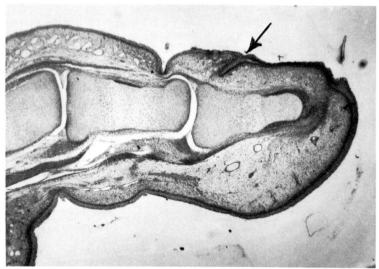

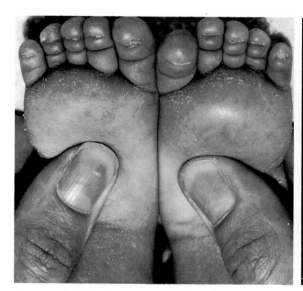

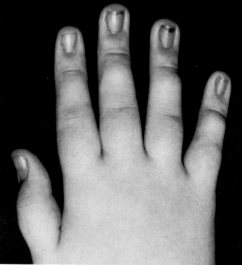

Figure 4–27. Fetal lymphedema may distort the form of the nails, as exemplified in a newborn (left) and a child (right) with peripheral lymphedema as one feature of the XO Turner syndrome. The narrow, hyperconvex nails with the appearance of a deep-set nail base are the residual consequences of prior lymphedema.

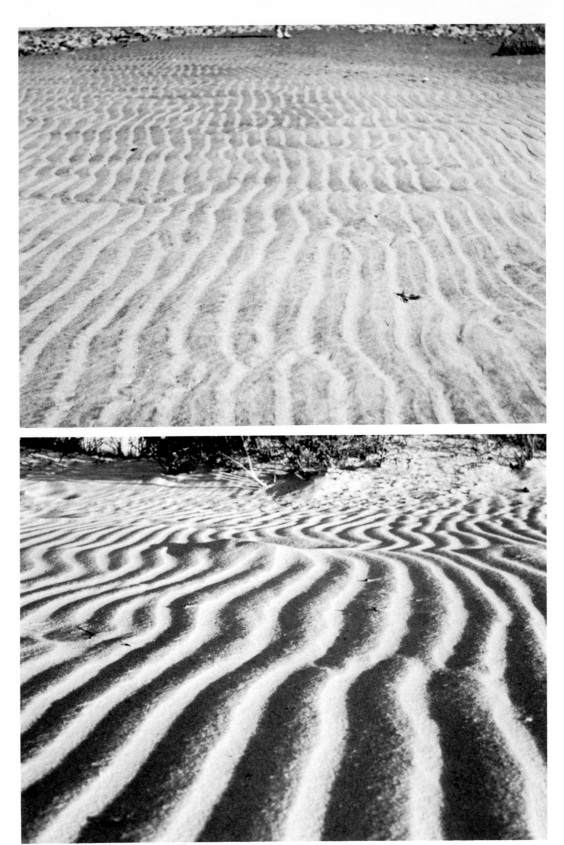

Figure 4–28. The ridges in the sand were generated at right angles to the direction of flow of water (above) and wind (below). Where there are undulations in the surface, the forces generate curvilinear patterns. Dermal ridges seem to be determined in somewhat similar fashion, tending to be at right angles to the direction of growth stretch.

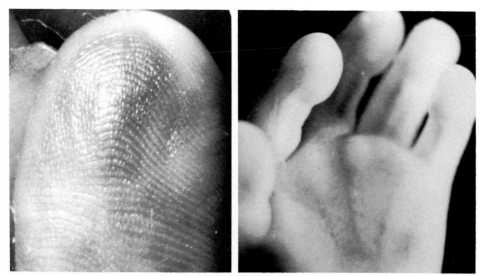

Figure 4–29. The dermal ridges, shown here on the distal finger of an infant (left) tend to develop at right angles to the growth stretch exerted on the skin by the development of the underlying tissues. Where there are pads, such as those shown in the fingertips and interdigital areas of the palm of a 10-week fetus (right), these result in the development of curvilinear ridge patterns, such as the low arch pattern on the fingertip shown to the left.

of the brain would appear to be of fundamental genetic determination. The growth of the brain in size (magnitude) and shape (direction) exerts a major mechanical impact on the form of the tissues that surround and relate to the brain in the craniofacial region. The early neural structures have the predominant impact. Thus, the brain affects the

development of the calvarium and its sutures,[16] the optic cup evagination from the brain sets the stage for the orbit,[17] the invaginating neural olfactory placodes are primarily responsible for the subsequent formation of the nose and its accessories, and the inva-

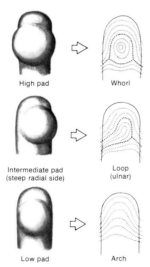

Figure 4–30. The fingertip dermal ridge patterning appears to relate to the form of the fingertip pads at the time of development of the dermal ridges. (From Mulvihill, J. J., and Smith, D. W.: Genesis of dermatoglyphics. J. Pediatr. 75:579, 1969.)

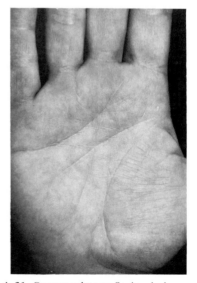

Figure 4–31. Creases relate to flexional planes of folding, always being secondary to mechanical forces. The upper palmar crease relates to the sloping plane of folding of the third, fourth, and fifth metacarpal-phalangeal joints, the thenar crease relates to the flexion of the thenar region, and the mid-palmar crease represents the folding plane between these two.

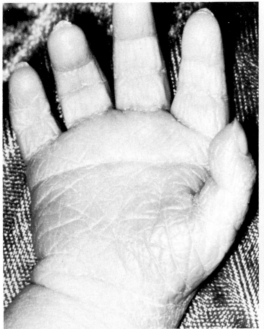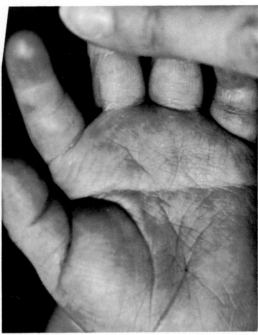

Figure 4–32. Minor differences in the form of the hand can result in a single crease across the upper palm (simian crease). The hand to the left has a short fifth finger and a single crease as a consequence. It also has an absence of the thenar crease (seen in the hand on the right), indicating a past functional deficit in oppositional flexional folding of the thenar region. The fine little creases occur when the skin of the hand is thin and have no further relevance.

ginating auditory placode forms the inner ear and is responsible for much of the orientation of the temporal wing of the sphenoid bone. Therefore, the statement that the "face reflects the brain" has much to support it. Particular features in the craniofacial region are summarized below.

Figures 4–33 and 4–34 emphasize the integral relationship that exists between the face and the brain. Beyond the mechanical impacts of brain development on facial form there are indirect effects of neuromuscular function on facial form. Such effects are depicted in Figures 4–35 and 4–36.

The Calvarium. It is the growth and shape of the brain that normally set the form of the calvarium. Thus, in the absence of problems of calvarial development, such as constraint molding and/or craniostenosis, it is the brain that determines the shape of the calvarium. For example, a narrow forehead means a narrow forebrain, and a brachycephalic skull means a shorter length of brain.

The organ capsule of the brain, the dura mater, is literally the mother tissue in the development of the bony calvarium and its sutures (Fig. 4–37). The calvarium consists of bony plates joined by strips of unminer-

alized dura, the sutures. These suture sites relate directly to the form of the early brain. As the brain grows outward, it balloons out the overlying dura mater. The brain is not a smooth hemisphere, and dural reflections occur into the recesses of the brain. The dural reflections are shown in Figure 4–38. Overlying these dural reflections, there is normally no ossification as long as there is continued growth stretch, as shown in Figure 4–39.[16] These are the sites of the sutures.[16] The metopic and sagittal sutures relate to the sites of the dural reflection into the interhemispheral fissure, the falx cerebri. The lambdoid sutures relate to the sites of the dural reflection between the cerebrum and cerebellum, the falx cerebelli. The coronal suture relates to the insular sulcus of the brain with its dural reflection off the sphenoid wing, which faithfully fills in this sulcus in the brain.[16]

Between the sites of dural reflection, ossification begins within the membranous dura. These niduses of ossification spread outward toward the sites of the patient sutures, as shown in Figure 4–39. The radial orientation of the ossification appears to relate to the tensile forces. At the sites of initial ossification

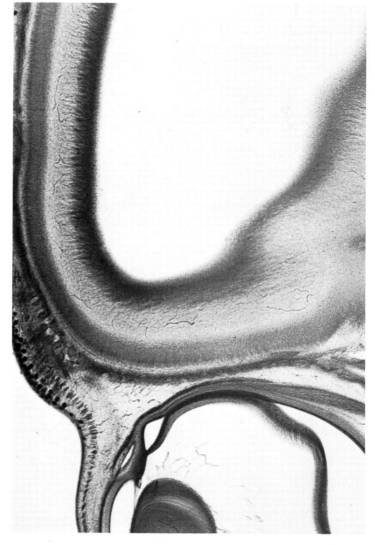

Figure 4–33. At 10 weeks, the cerebrum, which has only one cortical layer at this stage, is molding the forehead. The upper face is influenced by the early brain derivatives, the eyes. The mesenchymal tissues will soon condense and organize the supportive skeletal framework in accordance with these neural tissues. The growth of the cranial base anterior to the pituitary will occur in relationship to the frontal growth of the brain.

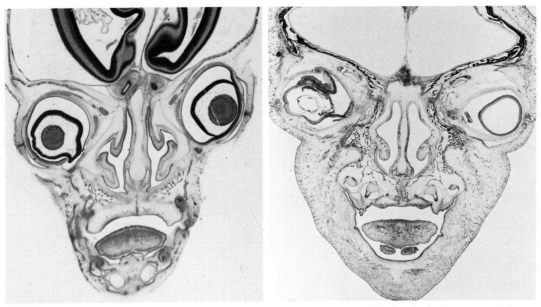

Figure 4–34. At 11 weeks (left) the relationship between the brain (contracted by fixation), the eyes, and the now cartilaginous upper facial skeleton is beautifully evident. This is also evident at 20 weeks (right, with brain removed), by which time much of the non-midline facial skeleton is ossified. Note the continuity between the cranial base and the facial skeleton. The anterior base of the brain *is* the roof of the face. (Left, from the Armed Forces Institute of Pathology, negative #76-5996. Right, from Burdi, A. R.: Early development of the human basicranium. Symposium on Development of the Basicranium. Edited by Bosma, J. F., NIDR; DHEW Publication No. (NIH) 77-989, Bethesda, MD, 1977.)

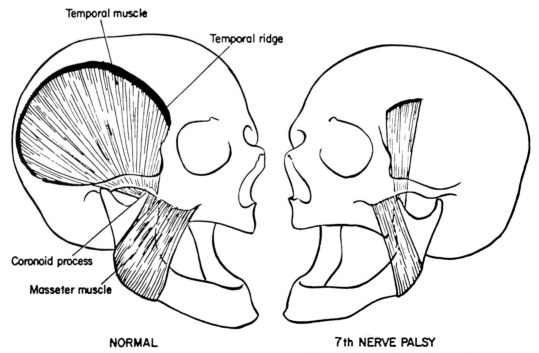

Figure 4–35. Mechanical force relationships between function and form as illustrated in a 60-year-old man who had a unilateral seventh nerve palsy from early in life. On the affected side the facial muscles were quite small, and all the sites of muscle attachment were less prominent on the affected side.

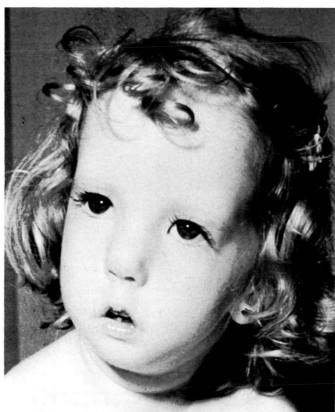

Figure 4–36. This girl is lacking sixth and seventh nerve function, a problem referred to as Moebius malformation sequence. The facial impact is *secondary* to the longstanding deficit of forces in the developing face. The almond-shaped eye is interpreted as being secondary to a deficiency of orbicularis oculi function, the small alae nasae to a deficit in the muscles that attach to this cartilage, and the small mouth to a lack of orbicularis oris muscle function. The shallow temporal region is ascribed to weakness of the temporal muscle, the shallow malar region to deficit of masseter function, and the small mandible to a diminished function of the mandible.

in the calvarium there may be small external promontories, most evident in infancy and childhood. These may be noted toward the center of each frontal bone, each parietal

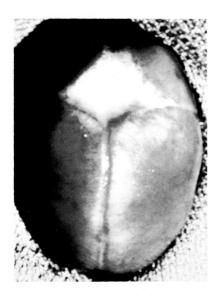

Figure 4–37. The calvarium in a 20-week fetus showing anterior fontanel and sutures.

bone, and each lateral portion of the occipital bone. They appear to be normal features. The major era in the early development of the calvarium is from 12 to 16 weeks.

In areas of the developing calvarium where the stretch forces may be less concise, such as in the region of the parietal bone near the posterior fontanel, multiple small centers of ossification may develop and then coalesce. These are referred to as wormian bones.

The implication that it is the early brain form that determines the sites of dural reflection and thereby the location of sutures is supported by aberrations of early brain morphogenesis that give rise to altered dural reflections and thereby to variance in the sutures of the calvarium.[16] Examples are shown in Figures 4–40 and 4–41.

There are several means by which the sutures of the calvarium may be altered. These include primary defects of brain, problems in suture development, metabolic problems, and external constraint.[18]

A serious deficit of brain growth, with a lack of stretch at suture lines, whether in primary microcephaly or in a shunted hydro-

Parietal bone

Posterior
fontanel and
lambdoidal
suture

Lateral venous
sinus

Occipital bone

Tentorium
cerebelli

Falx cerebri
attachment to
crista galli

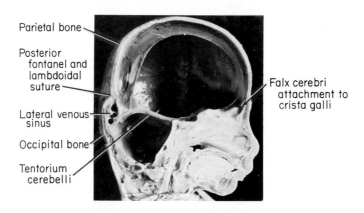

Crista galli, site of attachment of the falx cerebri

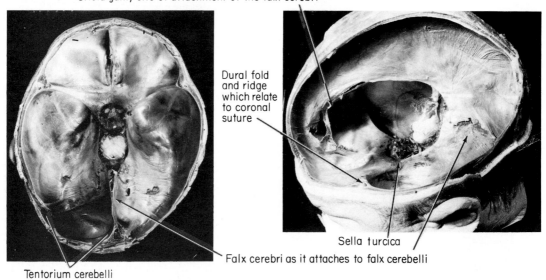

Dural fold
and ridge
which relate
to coronal
suture

Sella turcica

Tentorium cerebelli

Falx cerebri as it attaches to falx cerebelli

Figure 4–38. The dural reflections, which relate mechanically to the recesses in the developing brain, are shown above at 16 weeks and below in a term baby. Note how the lines of growth stretch are evident in the alignment of collagen fibrils within the dura. (From Professors Töndury and Kubik, University of Zurich.)

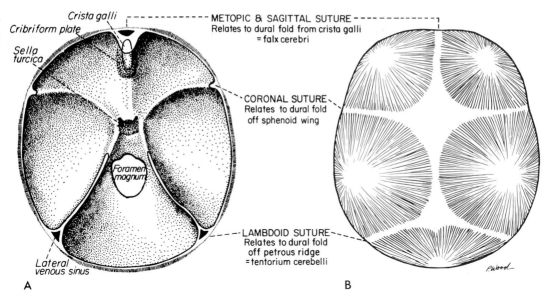

Figure 4–39. Conceptual drawing from a 17-week fetus, by which time the early calvarium is formed. The basilar view (left) shows the sites of dural reflection from the crista galli, sphenoid wings, and petrous ridges. These dural reflections are the sites of passive sutural development, as shown to the right. The top view of the early calvarium shows how ossification begins in the central spots between the dural reflections and spreads centrifugally toward the sutures. (From Smith, D. W., and Töndury, G.: Origins of the calvarium and its sutures. Am. J. Dis. Child. *132*:662, 1978.)

cephalus, may allow for mineralization at one or more of the suture lines. This secondary craniostenosis may then lead to further problems.

A primary defect of brain formation may affect the presence or site of dural reflections and hence the presence and sites of the sutures. One example is holoprosencephaly. A failure of diverticulation of the two cerebral vesicles will yield a single cerebral ventricle and no interhemispheral fissure. This is usually, but not always, accompanied by lack of a metopic suture.

External constraint of the developing fetal head may result in a lack of growth stretch at a given suture, resulting in craniosynostosis. This appears to be the most common mode of etiology for this problem.[18, 19]

The impact of the craniostenosis on craniofacial form will depend on the age of onset of craniostenosis and the suture(s) involved. Sagittal craniostenosis limits the lateral growth of the calvarium, resulting in a narrow, elongated, scaphocephalic head shape. Coronal stenosis limits the anterior-posterior growth, resulting in a short and wide brachy-

Figure 4–40. Conjoined twins provide an experiment of nature that demonstrates that the suture sites relate to the dural reflections. At the sites of juncture of the two brains there are dural reflections, and at these locations there are sutures and fontanels in positions where they would not normally be present. (From Smith, D. W., and Töndury, G.: Origins of the calvarium and its sutures. Am. J. Dis. Child. *132*:662, 1978.)

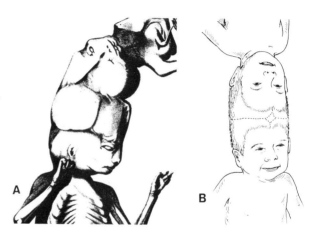

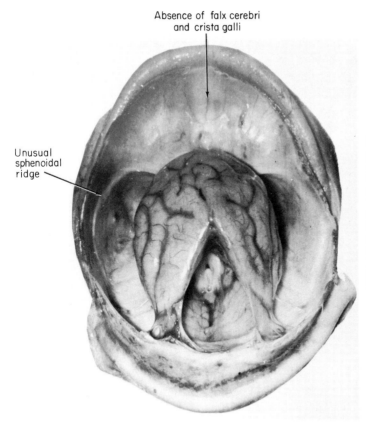

Absence of falx cerebri
and crista galli

Unusual
sphenoidal
ridge

Figure 4–41. An instance of alobar holo-prosencephaly. Because there was no in-terhemispheral fissure, there is no dural reflection at this site (falx cerebri), and as a consequence there is no metopic suture. There is also an aberrant alignment of the sphenoid wings relating to the altered brain impact in this location. This was associated wtih a comparable aberrant alignment of the coronal sutures. (From DeMeyer, W., White, P. T.: EEG in ho-loprosencephaly (arhinencephaly). Arch. Neurol. *11*:507–520, 1964.

cephalic head shape. Early coronal cranio-stenosis also prevents the forward growth of the brain and hence the anterior growth of the cranial base. Since the cranial base is the roof of the face, the midface tends to be retrusive. Also, the orbits become shallow, the eyes more widely spaced, and the fore-head high.

Craniostenosis of both the sagittal and co-ronal sutures will limit the capacity for brain growth and will usually cause increased intra-cranial pressure. Roentgenograms of the skull may show a beaten-silver appearance. This is at least partially due to a more vertical orientation of the bone fibrils within the calvarium, which tend to align in relation to the altered stress forces. The head tends to become tower-shaped, so-called oxycephaly, acrocephaly, or turricephaly.

The head is quite malleable, especially in fetal life. This is a normal and obviously necessary phenomenon during vaginal deliv-ery. During delivery the bony plates of the calvarium overlap at the sutures, sometimes to a surprising degree. Such molding is usu-ally transient, being limited to a few days.

Prolonged uterine constraint with com-pression of the fetal head during late fetal life may give rise to deformations of the head that only slowly resolve with time, or that may merit management in achieving a more normal resolution.[18]

The Cranial Base. The anterior cranial base develops from cartilage that becomes ossified, with persisting epiphysis-like growth centers posterior and anterior to the sella turcica. The region from the sella turcica anteriorly, which is designated as the anterior cranial base, tends to grow forward in ac-cordance with frontal brain growth. Hence, its growth follows that of neural growth, with 56 per cent completed by birth and 70 per cent completed by the age of two years.[16] It is important to appreciate that the anterior cranial base is the roof of the face from which the maxillary-ethmoid complex projects downward, and the anterior portion is the nasal bridge, as shown in Figure 4–33.

A deficit of frontal brain growth may yield a shorter cranial base and a less prominent nasal bridge. A shorter cranial base will gen-erally yield a flatter facial profile with a tendency toward a smaller and retrusive mid-face.

Eyes. The early outpouchings from the diencephalon, the optic cups, induce the formation of a lens in the overlying ectoderm: thus begins the formation of the eye. Surrounding mesenchymal cells condense to form the globular eye capsule within which the collagen fibrils align in relation to the fluid pressure from within the eye. Around the eye the mesenchymal tissues condense to form the bony orbit, which conforms to and is shaped in relation to the eye.[17]

A problem of fluid mechanics within the eye may result in increased pressure (glaucoma). This tends to distort the shape of the tense eye toward greater anterior globular prominence. It may also result in cloudiness of the cornea and destructive changes within the eye leading to eventual blindness.

A small eye (microphthalmia) will yield a small orbit. A lack of any optic cup will yield *no* orbit.[17] The accessory tissues of muscles, lacrimal apparatuses, eyebrows, eyelids, and eyelashes all relate to the development of the early optic evagination.[17] For example, an altered position of the early orbit is accompanied by predictable secondary development of all these accessory structures in the aberrant position of the optic vesicle, as exemplified in Figure 4–42.

Ears. *Inner Ear:* The otic placode, which is neural type tissue, invaginates from the surface ectoderm to become the otocyst. The differential growth of the otocyst leads to the beautiful spiral of the cochlea and the form of the vestibular apparatus. The mesenchyme around the otic placode is induced to form cartilage that faithfully conforms to its shape and that exerts a major role in the development of the sphenoid wing.

Middle Ear: The derivatives of the second and third branchial arches form the malleus, incus, and stapes as a connecting functional link between the eardrum and the round window of the cochlea, thus transmitting the vibrations to the cochlea. Any ankylosis within the joints of these bones may result in a problem of conductive deafness.

External Ear: The external auricle forms from the cartilaginous cores of the early hillocks of Hiss, which blend into a sheet of cartilage that grows throughout life. Mild to moderate deformations of the external auricle are common in the newly born baby, relating to constraint of the pliable auricle in

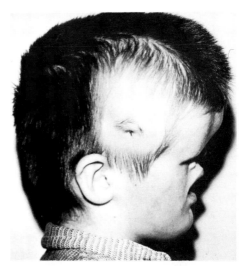

Figure 4–42. A rudimentary eye projected to an unusual temporal location in this individual. At this site the early optic vesicle mechanically gave rise to the development of a small optic cup. Furthermore, there was the development of periocular muscles, lacrimal apparatus, and eyelids, plus the growth of the hair at the eyebrow location and a zone of periocular hair growth suppression. (From Smith, D. W., and Gong, B. T.: Scalp-hair patterning: Its origin and significance relative to early brain and upper facial development. Teratology 9:17, 1974.)

late fetal life. Oligohydramnios accentuates such deformation and may result in an "accordioned" ear, an ear that is flattened against the calvarium, or other changes. The shoulder may be pressed up under the auricle in such situations as breech presentation, resulting in uplifting of the lower auricle. These distortions tend to resolve toward normal form after birth and are thoroughly benign deformations. Localized compression that affects one ear more than the other may result in overgrowth of the compressed ear.[20]

A distended jugular lymph sac, such as frequently occurs in the XO Turner fetus, may distort the auricle, making it more prominent and slanted than usual.[10]

The position and form of the cartilaginous folds of the auricle relate largely to the sites of insertion and origin of the auricular muscles.[21] Thus, defects of form of the external auricle may be the consequence of aberration in development and/or function of particular ear muscles. For example, absence of the posterior auricular ear muscle, which normally holds the ear in toward the calvarium, results in a protruding auricle (see Figs. 4–43 and 4–44), while absence of the superior

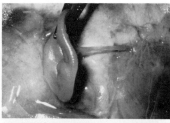

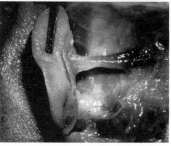

Figure 4–43. The posterior auricular muscle attaches from the concha of the ear to the mastoid region, thus holding the auricle toward the head. The upper photo is from a 16-week fetus and the lower a 20-week fetus. (From Smith, D. W., and Takashima, H.: Protruding auricle: A neuromuscular sign. Lancet *1*:747, 1978.)

auricular ear muscle results in a folded-over "lop" ear that may appear low in placement (Figs. 4–45 and 4–46). The inner conchal plical folds appear to relate to the intrinsic auricular ear muscles, and defects in their

development may result in varying degrees of a simple form to the concha. Experimental studies in the rodent have shown that early denervation of the seventh nerve, which supplies the auricular ear muscles, will result in a simple auricle that lacks the usual conchal folds.

Nose and Nasopharynx. The neural olfactory pit invaginates from the surface ectoderm and then sends its axons to synapse with those of the olfactory lobes. Later, when the base of the skull becomes cartilage and bone, these axons create the sites of "perforation" in the cribriform plate. Around the edges of the olfactory pit, the median and lateral nasal swellings rapidly grow out and coalesce with the maxillary swelling, to form much of the external nose and to fuse inferiorly to form the upper lip. The invaginating olfactory pits meet posteriorly with the foregut, and the epithelium between them breaks down, providing ready communication between the nasal and oral cavities. The cartilaginous nasal septum is in direct continuity with the anterior base of the skull, and hence alterations in growth of the base of the skull may secondarily affect nasal morphogenesis. Fusion of the maxillary palatal shelves with the nasal septum separates the nasal cavity from the mouth proper. Cartilaginous plates

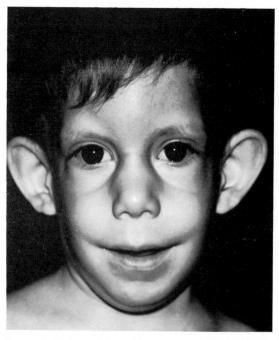

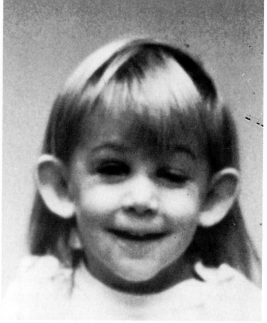

Figure 4–44. Left, A boy with neuromuscular weakness who had protruding ears as one feature. Right, A girl with XO Turner syndrome who has protruding ears plus unilateral ptosis of the eyelid. The protruding ears are a secondary mechanical neuromuscular sign, as is the ptosis of the eyelid. For each, the question is raised whether the primary problem is neurological or muscular. (From Smith, D. W., and Takashima, H.: Protruding auricle: A neuromuscular sign. Lancet *1*:747, 1978.)

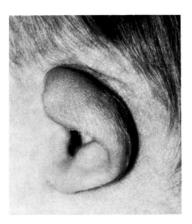

Figure 4–45. Lop ear, a secondary deformation due to a defect in development of function of the superior auricular ear muscle, which attaches the superior auricle to the head.

develop in the ala nasi, and these have muscle attachments that allow for constriction of the nares. Within the nose the cartilaginous turbinates grow, and evaginations from the nasal cavity occur into the surrounding bone. These evaginations, the sinuses, aerate the surrounding bones. This substantially reduces their weight while still providing excellent structural support. Sinus development is largely incomplete at birth. The first pharyngeal pouch persists as the eustachian tube and middle ear. Evaginations from the middle ear aerate the mastoid portion of the temporal bone, in similar fashion to the sinuses.

Late uterine constraint may distort the nose. Most commonly it may be compressed to one side. After birth this usually resolves

Figure 4–46. Summary of relationship between the extrinsic ear muscles and ear form. (Courtesy of Thomas Stebbins, University of Washington School of Medicine.)

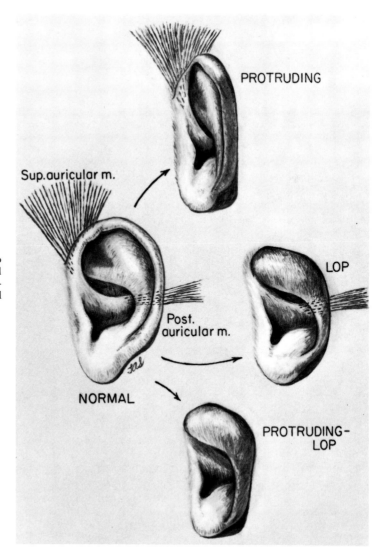

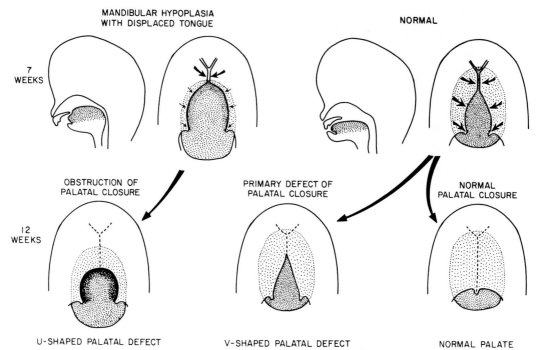

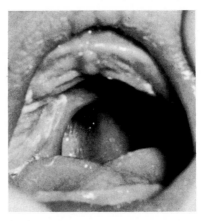

Figure 4–47. Pathways leading to defects of palatal closure as viewed in the lateral aspect and from above the palate. The left side lingual obstruction to closure of normal palatine shelves because of a small mandible with retroplaced tongue. This leads to a U-shaped palatal defect. The right side shows the normal closure of the palatine shelves and the V-shaped palatine defect that results from a primary problem in their closure. (From Hanson, J. W., and Smith, D. W.: U-shaped palatal defect in the Robin anomalad: Developmental and clinical relevance. J. Pediatr. *87*:30, 1975.)

spontaneously, though some manual pulling and remolding may be merited. Persisting compression may limit the growth of the nose, as in a face presentation. However, postnatal catch-up growth will usually result in a restoration to normal form.

As previously mentioned, aberrations of the growth of the cranial base, such as occur with problems of frontal brain growth, may alter both the relative position of the nasal bridge and the position and form of the nose.

Problems with the development and/or function of the musculature of the ala nasi may result in a narrow nose with small alar wings.

The sinuses tend to extend well into the solid bone that surround them. If there is a loss of permanent teeth from the upper jaw, the maxillary sinus will extend further than usual, coming into close proximity with the alveolar ridge at the sites of the missing teeth.

Palate and Tongue. The palatal shelves, which are initially projecting downward alongside the tongue, undergo a shift into the horizontal position and then fuse from front to back with each other and with the nasal septum. If the mandible is unusually small, there may be posterior displacement

of the tongue, which will tend to occlude closure of the palatal shelves, giving rise to a U-shaped palatal defect,[22] as shown in Figures 4–47 through 4–49. The posteriorly displaced tongue may obstruct the posterior

Figure 4–48. Robin sequence with U-shaped palatal defect secondary to interposition of the retroplaced tongue, itself the consequence of a small mandible. Note that the retroplaced tongue has allowed the development of prominent rugous ridging in the anterior portion of the palate. (From Hanson, J. W., and Smith, D. W.: U-shaped palatal defect in the Robin anomalad: Developmental and clinical relevance. J. Pediatr. *87*:30, 1975.)

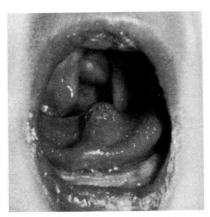

Figure 4–49. U-shaped palatal defect with molding of the tongue, which apparently remained partially interposed between the palatal shelves from early in development.

pharynx, giving rise to partial upper airway obstruction at birth. The initiating problem in mandibular size may be a malformation, and hence the consequences are termed the early micrognathia *malformation* sequence, or the Robin *malformation* sequence. The small mandible might also be the result of early fetal constraint with limitation of mandibular growth; in this instance the diagnosis would tend toward early micrognathia *deformation* sequence.

Not only does the tongue play a significant mechanical role in palatal closure but it also exerts a major impact on palatal form. Normally there are lateral palatine ridges that extend down from the roof of the palate between the alveolar ridges and the central palate, as shown in Figure 4–50.[23] These ridges are prominent in fetal life and are composed of mucopolysaccharide-rich connective tissue and myriads of small salivary glands. The force of the tongue thrust tends to smooth them out during fetal life. Any disorder that limits tongue thrust into the palate, such as hypotonia, other neurologic deficits, or microglossia, will cause prominent lateral palatine ridges (Fig. 4–50), often giving the appearance of a "narrow, high-arched" palate. At the other extreme, an enlarged tongue may result in relative flattening and even broadening of the hard palate. Thus the tongue, a very strong muscle, exerts a major impact within the mouth.

A narrow palate that appears highly arched not uncommonly develops in children with mental deficiency (Fig. 4–51). The reason for this is not clear, but it may relate to a deficit

in functional usage of the facial musculature. A narrow palate may also develop in patients with coronal suture craniostenosis.

Alveolar Ridge, Teeth, and Mandible. The tooth anlagen develop as ectodermal downgrowths that interact with the underlying mesenchyme to form the teeth, which then erupt, usually through the channel of their original downgrowth. If there is a failure of tooth development the alveolar ridge lacks prominence at that region. Thus the major mass of the alveolar ridges relates to the teeth. The form of the enamel crown of a tooth, which is produced by the ectodermal component, is genetically determined and allows for amazing interdigitation between the upper and lower teeth. The forces of biting and chewing tend to foster alignment of the teeth. The growth of the lower jaw—the mandible—tends to follow the lead of the upper jaw. This applies to lateral growth as well. Thus, if the maxilla is narrow, the mandible will also tend to be narrow. However, a deficit of function of the mandible will tend to slow its growth rate.

The muscles of the mandible are powerful, and their sites of attachment give rise to bony promontories. Figure 4–35 shows the impact of a unilateral facial nerve palsy on these muscles and therefore on the bony form of the face. The impact of the facial muscles on bony promontories is dramatically exemplified by experimental studies in rodents. For example, early resection of the masseter muscle results in a complete lack of the coronoid process, its site of insertion on the mandible (Fig. 4–52).

If the teeth are crowded, one or more may erupt in an aberrant alignment. Usually the easiest management is removal of the tooth that is "crowded out." Malalignment of the teeth is not uncommon. Orthodontic methods of constraint have become a common practice in realignment of the teeth and jaws during childhood.

Thorax and Lung. The growth of the ribs and the thoracic cage is integral to the full development of the lungs. The lungs develop as a progressive arborization from an outbudding of the foregut. The septation of the thoracic and abdominal cavities by the diaphragm allows the fetus to make respiratory movements. The full growth of the thoracic cage is important during the latter phase of lung development when the lung progresses from a solid organ tissue to one with alveolar

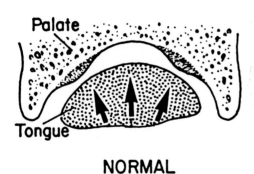

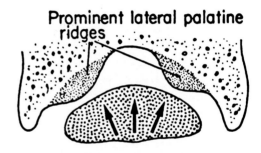

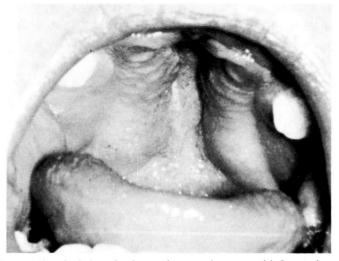

Figure 4–50. Above, Cross section depiction of palate and tongue in a normal infant and one in whom there was a deficit of tongue thrust into the hard palate, which allowed for the development of prominent lateral palatal ridges. Below, Prominent lateral palatine shelves between the alveolar ridges and the center of the palate in this hypotonic infant indicated that the hypotonia was of long standing.

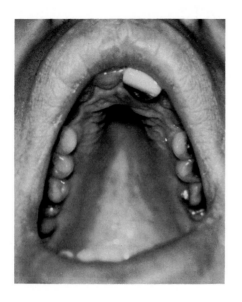

Figure 4–51. Narrow palate in a mentally retarded adult, the presumed consequences of the deficiency of normal forces relative to the growth and form of the maxilla. Such a narrow palate is unusual in mentally retarded infants but not in retarded older children.

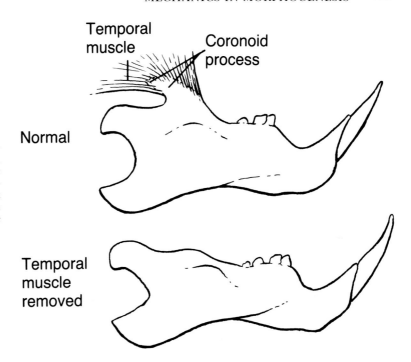

Figure 4–52. Early postnatal removal of the masseter muscle in the rat results in a lack of the coronoid process of the mandible, the bony protuberance that normally results from the tension of the masseter muscle at this site of attachment.

sacs capable of aeration. Restrictive crowding during the late fetal lung growth may result in the lung being incompletely developed by birth, and the infant will have respiratory insufficiency at birth. Deficit of lung growth may be due to a number of causes, as summarized in Table 4–3. External constraint of an unusual degree, such as a bicornuate uterus, may be a cause. With oligohydramnios, the constraint to thoracic growth is frequently sufficient to impair full lung development.[24] As a consequence, respiratory insufficiency is the predominant cause of death in newborn babies affected by oligohydramnios. Crowding of the lung during growth may be intrinsic, as in diaphragmatic hernia. A diaphragmatic "hernia," of course, represents incomplete development of the diaphragm. This allows variable amounts of abdominal contents to gain access to the thoracic cage and limits the capacity for full lung growth. Hence, the newly born baby with a diaphragmatic hernia may die of respiratory insufficiency, even if an excellent diaphragmatic repair with removal of abdominal contents from the thoracic cage is done soon after birth.

The thoracic cage is rather malleable and may show alterations of form in relation to constraint. If the fetus is in a position with the chin forced into the chest, for example, there may be both a small mandible and a mild "impression" on the chest wall.

Cardiovascular. The early heart ducts fuse to become one tube, which then undergoes almost a figure-eight type of contortion to become the four-chambered heart. Growth of specific ridges within the convoluting

Table 4–3. **CAUSES OF INADEQUATE LATE FETAL LUNG GROWTH**

	General	Examples
EXTERNAL CONSTRAINT	Oligohydramnios	Renal agenesis Chronic leakage of amniotic fluid
	Small uterine cavity	Bicornuate uterus Large uterine fibroid(s)
INTRINSIC CONSTRAINT	Limited thoracic growth	Thoracic asphyxiant dystrophy
	Thoracic mass	Diaphragmatic hernia

heart-to-be gives rise to separation of the blood channels and development of the valves. Thus, the growth of the atrioventricular cushions assists in the separation of the atria and ventricles and the formation of the tricuspid and mitral valves, whereas the growth of the conotruncal pads separates the single outlet truncus into the aorta and pulmonary arteries with the development of aortic and pulmonary valves. Throughout cardiac morphogenesis the direction and force of the streams of blood play a major role in the development of cardiac form. For example, the blood coming from the placenta through the ductus venosus flows across the right atrium and maintains the patency of the foramen ovale, directly shunting the blood into the left atrium. As soon as the large placental flow ceases at birth and other changes take place, such as closure of the ductus arteriosus and the "opening up" of the pulmonary vascular bed, the direction and magnitude of blood flow change in such a manner that the foramen ovale closes.

Any anatomic change in early heart development usually has a major effect on subsequent cardiac morphogenesis by changing the biomechanics within the developing heart. For example, a ventricular septal defect will result in excessive shunting of blood into the right ventricle and the pulmonary system, thus resulting in enlargement of the right ventricle. The excessive pressure on the pulmonary circulation will eventually cause increased vascular resistance, further increasing the load on the right ventricle, which may then begin to fail in its function. Early intervention, with closure of the ventricular septal defect, may prevent such biomechanical consequences, all of which may be interpreted as *deformations* in the cardiovascular system.

Interference with the early flow patterns may be the primary cause of problems in cardiac morphogenesis. Ishikawa[25] produced defects of the heart and great vessels in 42 per cent of chick embryos by placing them in a centrifuge for nine hours during the period of cardiac morphogenesis. The cardiac defects were presumed to be the consequence of the alterations in the flow patterns during this critical time in heart development. Similar alterations in chick heart morphogenesis have been induced by Clark, utilizing mechanical alterations in early vascular flow patterns.[26]

The peripheral blood vessels develop as a coalescence of multiple small lacunae into vessels. Initially there tends to be a general network of small vessels. The magnitude and direction of flow will result in enlargement of some of these minute vessels in a particular direction, whereas a diminished flow will result in regression of vessels. Hence the vascularity develops to a major extent in relation to the needs of the region and to its form. If there is hypoplasia in a region, the vascular channels in that region will generally be smaller than usual.

Intestines. The endoderm outpouches in a forward direction as the foregut and posteriorly as the hindgut. As the intestine enlarges it extends beyond the abdominal wall into the allantoic sac and then returns later into the abdominal cavity. Its enlargement gives rise to multiple foldings in the gut and to overall rotation of the midgut so that the cecum ends up in the right lower quadrant. The capsule of the intestine—the peritoneum—follows this rotation and then becomes fixed to the inner abdominal wall at certain points. An incomplete rotation of the gut will result in unusual mesenteric attachments and will increase the liability toward volvulus of the midgut.

Any obstruction of the intestine will alter mechanics within the gut, giving rise to distention of the proximal gut and changes in the bowel wall. The distal segment, with less distention, will be unusually small in caliber.

Urinary Tract and Kidneys. The early mesonephric ridge has a longitudinal series of nephron elements that drain into a common mesonephric duct. Toward the lower end of this duct an outpouching occurs—the ureteral bud. This induces the formation of glomeruli and nephron elements in the adjacent metanephric blastema. The ureteral bud progressively arborizes, and each new bud induces a new group of glomeruli and nephrons, which communicate with the ureteral buds. The ureteral bud becomes the ureter, and its multiple branches become the collecting ducts and distal tubules. The induced elements become the glomeruli and the proximal renal tubules. If there is any obstruction to the flow of urine, which begins by eight to nine weeks in the human, the area proximal to the obstruction will become dilated. If the flow from a whole kidney is obstructed, the pelvic drainage system of the kidney becomes dilated; this is termed hydronephrosis. If it occurs during early development it may adversely affect renal morphogenesis, resulting in hypoplasia and the formation of "cysts" in the kidney. These are not true cysts; rather, they are dilations in the tubules that may appear as cysts on histologic sections of the kidney. Early obstruction to urine flow in the urethra results in the urethral obstruction malformation sequence, a series of consequences of the biomechanical effects of obstruction within the urinary tract.[11]

Any renal system disorder that results in a lack of urine flow into the amniotic space will usually cause a deficit of amniotic fluid during late fetal life. It does not matter whether the lack of urine is due to renal agenesis, hydronephrosis, or severe urethral obstruction, the consequences are the same—the oligohydramnios deformation sequence.

References

1. Thompson, D.: On Growth and Form. A New Edition. Cambridge, The University Press, 1942.
2. Dingwall, E. J.: Artificial Cranial Deformation: A Contribution to the Study of Ethnic Mutilation. London, John Bale, Sons and Danielsson, Ltd., 1931.
3. Dunn, P. M.: Growth retardation of infants with congenital postural deformities. Acta Med. Auxol. 7:63, 1975.
4. Hafez, E. S. E.: Reproductive failure in domestic mammals. In Benirschke, K. (ed.): Comparative Aspects of Reproductive Failure. New York, Springer-Verlag, 1967, pp. 44–95.
5. Smith, G. E.: The causation of the symmetrical thinning of the parietal bones in ancient Egyptians. J. Anat. Physiol. London 41:232, 1906–7.
6. Drachman, D. B., and Coulombre, A. J.: Experimental clubfoot and arthrogryposis multiplex congenita. Lancet 2:523, 1962.
7. Jago, R. H.: Arthrogryposis following treatment of maternal tetanus with muscle relaxants. Arch. Dis. Child. 45:277, 1970.
8. Moessinger, A. C.: Fetal akinesia deformation sequence: An animal model. Pediatrics 72:857, 1983.
9. Smith, D. W.: Redundant skin folds in the infant: Their origin and relevance. J. Pediatr. 94:1021, 1979.
10. Graham, J. M., Jr., and Smith, D. W.: Dominantly inherited pterygium colli. J. Pediatr. 98:664, 1981.
11. Pagon, R. A., Smith, D. W., and Shepard, T. H.: Urethral obstruction malformation complex: A cause of abdominal muscle deficiency and the "prune belly." J. Pediatr. 95:900, 1979.
12. Stephan, M. J., Smith, D. W., Ponzi, J. W., and Alden, E. R.: Origin of scalp vertex aplasia cutis. J. Pediatr. 101:850, 1982.
13. Smith, D. W., and Gong, B. T.: Scalp hair patterning as a clue to early fetal brain development. J. Pediatr. 83:374, 1969.
14. Mulvihill, J. J., and Smith, D. W.: Genesis of dermatoglyphics. J. Pediatr. 75:579, 1969.
15. Popich, G. A., and Smith, D. W: The genesis and significance of digital and palmar hand creases: Preliminary report. J. Pediatr. 77:1017, 1960.
16. Smith, D. W., and Töndury, G.: Origins of the calvarium and its sutures. Am. J. Dis. Child. 132:662, 1978.
17. Jones, K. L., Higginbottom, M. C., and Smith, D. W.: The determining role of the optic vesicles in orbital and periocular development and placement. Pediatr. Res. 14:703, 1980.
18. Graham, J. M., Jr.: Alterations in head shape as a consequence of fetal head constraint. Sem. Perinatol. 7:257, 1983.
19. Graham, J. M., deSaxe, M., and Smith, D. W.: Sagittal craniostenosis: Fetal head constraint as one possible cause. J. Pediatr. 95:747, 1979.
20. Aase, J. M.: Structural defects as a consequence of late intrauterine constraint: Craniotabes, loose skin, and asymmetric ear size. Sem. Perinatol. 7:270, 1983.
21. Smith, D. W., and Takashima, H.: Protruding auricle: A neuromuscular sign. Lancet 1:747, 1978.
22. Hanson, J. W., and Smith, D. W.: U-shaped palatal defect in the Robin anomalad: Developmental and clinical relevance. J. Pediatr. 87:30, 1975.
23. Hanson, J. W., Smith, D. W., and Cohen, M. M., Jr.: Prominent lateral palatine ridges: Developmental and clinical relevance. J. Pediatr. 89:54, 1976.
24. Thomas, I. T., and Smith, D. W.: Oligohydramnios, cause of the non-renal features of Potter's syndrome, including pulmonary hypoplasia. J. Pediatr. 84:811, 1974.
25. Ishikawa, Prof., Tokyo University Medical School. Personal communication.
26. Clark, E. B.: Functional aspects of cardiac development. In Zak, R. (ed.): Growth of the Heart in Health and Disease. New York, Raven Press, 1984.

5

Concluding
Remarks

Ever since Peter Dunn acquainted us with the basic concepts of deformation we have been increasingly impressed by the frequency with which unusual mechanical forces may be deduced as being responsible for structural birth defects. The impact of mechanical forces on form not only has provided an understanding of the extrinsic constraint deformations but also has led to the appreciation that many of the malformation sequences can be interpreted as an initiating malformation that gave rise to altered mechanical forces and a cascade of intrinsic deformation. Furthermore, this mechanical perspective provides a better understanding of factors in normal morphogenesis.

The major emphasis of this text has been on the extrinsic constraint deformations that are secondary to crowding in utero. These should, to the extent possible, be distinguished from malformations with or without secondary intrinsic deformation. Not only are there major differences in the etiology, prognosis, management, and recurrence risk counsel, but there also is a profound difference in the attitude that can be conveyed to the parents. The child with extrinsic deformation can usually be interpreted as normal, and the parents can look forward to the restoration of normal form. This attitude toward considering extrinsic deformations as a separable category of birth defects is also critical in providing better answers relative to

etiology and prevention. The etiologic factors that may cause extrinsic deformation are obviously very different from those that cause malformation problems. The preventive measures for extrinsic deformations are also different and entail such considerations as the controversial external version for malposition in utero and the surgical reconstruction of a malformed uterus. Furthermore, since extrinsic deformations are more common in infants of primigravida mothers and in larger fetuses, it is quite reasonable to anticipate that the incidence of extrinsic deformations might increase as a consequence of smaller families and larger babies.

The basic principles of extrinsic deformation are simple. The magnitude and direction of force have their impact on form. The same simple precepts are relevant to the reformational management. With rare exception this may be accomplished by rational application of subtle forces.

Why has it taken such a long time for this knowledge to become an integral part of medicine? It is not because extrinsic deformations are rare—they are common. It is not because the concepts are new—they are old. Possibly one reason is that the overall concepts that relate to the developmental pathology, diagnosis, and management of extrinsic deformations are so simple. In recent times there has been a tendency to look for more complex answers of a biochemical, molecular, or physiologic nature and to bypass the simple mechanistic approaches. Hence this book is dedicated to bringing the mechanical aspects of morphogenesis and deformation into the mainstream of medicine, where they belong.

Very few studies of extrinsic deformation in experimental animals have been done. One reason is that few creatures other than man tend to outgrow the uterus prior to birth and to have constraint deformations at birth. This is one price the slowly aging, rapidly growing, large-brained human must pay for his or her present level of evolvement.

Index

Page numbers in *italics* indicate illustrations.
Page numbers followed by (t) indicate tables.
Page numbers followed by *n* indicate notes.